Co-occurring Medical Illnesses in Child and Adolescent Psychiatry: Updates and Treatment Considerations

Editor

MATTHEW D. WILLIS

CHILD AND ADOLESCENT PSYCHIATRIC CLINICS OF NORTH AMERICA

www.childpsych.theclinics.com

Consulting Editor
TODD E. PETERS

January 2018 • Volume 27 • Number 1

ELSEVIER

1600 John F. Kennedy Boulevard • Suite 1800 • Philadelphia, Pennsylvania, 19103-2899

http://www.theclinics.com

CHILD AND ADOLESCENT PSYCHIATRIC CLINICS OF NORTH AMERICA Volume 27, Number 1
January 2018 ISSN 1056–4993, ISBN-13: 978-0-323-58186-8

Editor: Lauren Boyle
Developmental Editor: Kristen Helm

Child and Adolescent Psychiatric Clinics of North America (ISSN 1056-4993) is published quarterly by Elsevier Inc., 360 Park Avenue South, New York, NY 10010-1710. Months of issue are January, April, July, and October. Business and Editorial Offices: 1600 John F. Kennedy Boulevard, Suite 1800, Philadelphia, PA 19103-2899. Periodicals postage paid at New York, NY and additional mailing offices. Subscription prices are $322.00 per year (US individuals), $594.00 per year (US institutions), $100.00 per year (US students), $382.00 per year (Canadian individuals), $723.00 per year (Canadian institutions), $200.00 per year (Canadian students), $439.00 per year (international individuals), $723.00 per year (international institutions), and $200.00 per year (international students). International air speed delivery is included in all *Clinics* subscription prices. All prices are subject to change without notice. **POSTMASTER:** Send address changes to *Child and Adolescent Psychiatric Clinics of North America*, Elsevier Health Sciences Division, Subscription Customer Service, 3251 Riverport Lane, Maryland Heights, MO 63043. **Customer Service: 1-800-654-2452 (U.S. and Canada); 314-447-8871 (outside U.S. and Canada). Fax: 314-447-8029. E-mail:** JournalsCustomer Service-usa@elsevier.com **(for print support) or** journalsonlinesupport-usa@elsevier.com **(for online support).**

Reprints. For copies of 100 or more of articles in this publication, please contact the Commercial Reprints Department, Elsevier Inc., 360 Park Avenue South, New York, New York 10010-1710 Tel.: 212-633-3874; Fax: 212-633-3820, E-mail: reprints@elsevier.com.

Child and Adolescent Psychiatric Clinics of North America is covered in *MEDLINE/PubMed (Index Medicus), ISI, SSCI, Research Alert, Social Search, Current Contents,* and *EMBASE/Excerpta Medica.*

Contributors

CONSULTING EDITOR

TODD E. PETERS, MD, FAPA
Assistant Chief Medical Informatics Officer/Customer Relationship Manager, Vanderbilt University Medical Center, Associate Chief of Staff, Department of Psychiatry and Behavioral Sciences, Vanderbilt University Medical Center, Medical Director for Inpatient Services, Vanderbilt Psychiatric Hospital, Assistant Professor of Psychiatry and Behavioral Sciences, Vanderbilt University, Nashville, Tennessee

EDITOR

MATTHEW D. WILLIS, MD, MPH, FAAP
Attending Psychiatrist and Pediatrician, Hasbro Children's Partial Hospital Program, Assistant Professor (Clinical), Department of Psychiatry and Human Behavior, The Warren Alpert Medical School of Brown University, Rhode Island Hospital, Providence, Rhode Island, USA

AUTHORS

KRISTIN L. ANDERSON, MD, FAAP, FACP
Assistant Professor of Medicine and Pediatrics, Division of Pediatrics, Clinician Educator, The Warren Alpert Medical School of Brown University, Hasbro Children's Hospital, Rhode Island Hospital, Providence, Rhode Island, USA

CAROLINA CEREZO, MD
Associate Professor of Pediatrics, Pediatric Gastroenterology, The Warren Alpert Medical School of Brown University, Hasbro Children's Hospital, Providence, Rhode Island, USA

HEATHER A. CHAPMAN, MD
Pediatrician, Hasbro Children's Partial Hospital Program, Assistant Clinical Professor of Pediatrics, The Warren Alpert Medical School at Brown University, Providence, Rhode Island, USA

DIANE DERMARDEROSIAN, MD
Pediatric Director, Hasbro Children's Partial Hospital Program, Associate Clinical Professor of Pediatrics, The Warren Alpert Medical School at Brown University, Providence, Rhode Island, USA

JULIA L. DOSS, PsyD
Pediatric Psychologist, Residency Training Director, Department of Psychology, Minnesota Epilepsy Group, St Paul, Minnesota, USA

WILLIAM GALLENTINE, DO
Autoimmune Brain Disease Program, Associate Professor, Department of Pediatrics, Neurology Division, Duke University, Durham, North Carolina, USA

ARIS GARRO, MD, MPH
Associate Professor of Pediatrics and Emergency Medicine, Division of Pediatric Emergency Medicine, The Warren Alpert Medical School of Brown University, Rhode Island Hospital, Hasbro Children's Hospital, Providence, Rhode Island, USA

AMY GOLDBERG, MD, FAAP
Department of Pediatrics, The Warren Alpert Medical School of Brown University, Providence, Rhode Island, USA

LAURA C. HART, MD, MPH
Cecil G. Sheps Center for Health Services Research, Postdoctoral Fellow, The University of North Carolina at Chapel Hill, Chapel Hill, North Carolina, USA

MICHAEL HERZLINGER, MD
Assistant Professor of Pediatrics, Pediatric Gastroenterology, The Warren Alpert Medical School of Brown University, Hasbro Children's Hospital, Providence, Rhode Island, USA

MICHAEL P. KOSTER, MD
Clinician Educator, Associate Professor, Department of Pediatrics, The Warren Alpert Medical School of Brown University, Rhode Island Hospital, Hasbro Children's Hospital, Providence, Rhode Island, USA

NAVID MAHOOTI, MD, MPH
Clinical Instructor, Sports Medicine, North Shore Medical Center Internal Medicine Residency Program, North Shore Physicians Group, Mass General/North Shore Center, Danvers, Massachusetts, USA

GARY MASLOW, MD, MPH
Assistant Professor, Psychiatry and Behavioral Sciences, Duke University School of Medicine, Durham, North Carolina, USA

GENALYNNE C. MOONEYHAM, MD, MS
Autoimmune Brain Disease Program, Medical Instructor, Department of Pediatrics, Department of Psychiatry, Division of Child and Family Mental Health and Developmental Neurosciences, Duke University, Durham, North Carolina, USA

JESSICA MOORE, BA
Hasbro Children's Hospital, Providence, Rhode Island, USA

PAMELA J. MOSHER, MD, MDiv
Division of Child and Adolescent Psychiatry, The Hospital for Sick Children, Department of Supportive Care, Division of Psychosocial Oncology, Princess Margaret Cancer Centre, Assistant Professor, Department of Psychiatry, University of Toronto, Toronto, Ontario, Canada

SIGITA PLIOPLYS, MD
Head, Department of Child and Adolescent Psychiatry, Pediatric Neuropsychiatry Clinic, Ann & Robert H. Lurie Children's Hospital of Chicago, Professor of Psychiatry and Behavioral Sciences, Northwestern University, Chicago, Illinois, USA

CHRISTINA TORTOLANI, PhD
Assistant Professor, Department of Counseling, Educational Leadership and School Psychology, Rhode Island College, Adjunct Assistant Professor of Psychiatry and Human Behavior, The Warren Alpert Medical School at Brown University, Providence, Rhode Island, USA

HEATHER VAN MATER, MD, MS
Autoimmune Brain Disease Program, Assistant Professor, Department of Pediatrics, Rheumatology Division, Duke University, Durham, North Carolina, USA

MATTHEW D. WILLIS, MD, MPH, FAAP
Attending Psychiatrist and Pediatrician, Hasbro Children's Partial Hospital Program, Assistant Professor (Clinical), Department of Psychiatry and Human Behavior, The Warren Alpert Medical School of Brown University, Rhode Island Hospital, Providence, Rhode Island, USA

Contents

Eating disorders are a group of psychiatric disorders with potentially fatal medical complications. Early integrated care including the family as well as pediatric medicine, nutrition, psychology and psychiatry is critical for improving prognosis and limiting negative outcomes. Mental health services are a critical component of treatment; timely weight restoration maximizes efficacy. Despite being relatively common there are many misperceptions about eating disorders, their severity, and the associated morbidity and mortality. Opportunities exist within the medical and psychiatric communities for a better understanding of the complexity of diagnosing and treating patients with eating disorders.

Functional gastrointestinal disorders are very common. They result from dysfunctional interaction in the brain-gut axis. Although the nature is benign, symptoms may be debilitating. The etiology is multifactorial; therefore, the diagnosis should be approached in a biopsychosocial model. There are no biomarkers to characterize these conditions, but a solid understanding of the pathophysiology allows providers to present these disorders as a positive clinical diagnosis rather than a diagnosis of exclusion. Effective management entails close collaboration between the medical and mental health providers.

Lyme disease is endemic in parts of the United States, including New England, the Atlantic seaboard, and Great Lakes region. The presentation has various manifestations, many of which can mimic psychiatric diseases in children. Distinguishing manifestations of Lyme disease from those of psychiatric illnesses is complicated by inexact diagnostic tests and misuse of these tests when they are not clinically indicated. This article aims to describe manifestations of Lyme disease in children with an emphasis on Lyme neuroborreliosis. Clinical scenarios are presented and discussed. Finally, recommendations for clinical psychiatrists who encounter children with possible Lyme disease are presented.

Medical conditions that present with psychiatric symptoms are becoming increasingly well recognized in response to the emergence of the field of neuroimmunology. As the availability of testing for novel antineuronal antibodies has increased, so too has the clinical awareness of this diagnostic spectrum. Psychiatrists may have little exposure to this area of expertise, yet may be called on to assist in the diagnosis and treatment of patients with complex neuropsychiatric syndromes secondary to autoimmune encephalitis. This article summarizes the evaluation and management of patients with autoimmune encephalitis and describes emerging patterns in phenotype recognition.

Psychogenic nonepileptic seizures is a complicated biopsychosocial disorder with significant morbidity and high cost in children's social, emotional, family, and academic functioning as well as health care service utilization. Misdiagnosis and diagnostic delay, resulting from both lack of access to approved standards for diagnosing and service providers comfortable with diagnosing and treating this disorder, affect prognosis. Treatment in close proximity to symptom onset is thought to provide the best chance for remission.

Prevention and management of childhood obesity remains a public health priority and necessitates an integrated chronic care approach. Obesity prevention efforts should focus on healthy family-based lifestyle modifications. The United States Prevention Services Task Force recommends that children older than 6 years be screened for obesity and, if clinically indicated, be referred for moderate- to high-intensity comprehensive behavioral interventions. Childhood obesity and its comorbidities affect most medical specialties. A shared understanding of prevention strategies, lifestyle recommendations, screening guidelines for comorbidities, and stages of treatment will allow for more integrated and collaborative care.

Commercial sexual exploitation of children and child sex trafficking is a major public health issue globally. Domestic minor sex trafficking has become increasingly recognized within the United States. Sexually exploited minors are commonly identified as having psychosocial risk factors, including histories of abuse or neglect, running away, substance use or abuse, and involvement with child protective services. Youth also suffer a variety of physical and mental health consequences, including posttraumatic stress disorder, depression, anxiety, and suicidality. Child psychiatrists and other medical providers have the opportunity to identify, interact, and intervene on behalf of involved and at-risk youth.

Sports-related concussion (SRC) is a common problem in youth sports. Concussion may occur after a forceful hit to the body or head, resulting in transient neuropathologic changes that spontaneously resolve with relative rest and activity modification in most patients. Most SRCs are effectively managed by primary care physicians and sports medicine specialists. In some cases, symptoms may persist and the child and adolescent psychiatrist may be consulted. This article reviews important background information regarding SRC and highlights a variety of pharmacologic and nonpharmacologic treatment options that consultant psychiatrists should know.

Grief is ubiquitous in the experience of children and adolescents with illness but not always recognized or named, and as a result grief is not always treated effectively by child/adolescent psychiatrists or pediatricians. Grief can be misinterpreted or treated as stress, anxiety, depression, adolescent moodiness, or behavioral concerns. Pediatricians and child/adolescent psychiatrists are often insufficiently educated on the topic of grief.

More adolescents and young adults are surviving previously fatal childhood illness and need support to transition from pediatric care to adult-oriented care. There are many barriers, but guidelines and tools assist providers with emphasis on gradually addressing transition with patients and families. Child and adolescent psychiatrists should be particularly attuned to the needs of adolescents with previously identified mental illness who are at high risk of falling out of regular care during transition. Providers are also uniquely suited to address the needs of adolescents and young adults with intellectual and developmental disabilities.

Co-occurring Medical Illnesses in Child and Adolescent Psychiatry: Updates and Treatment Considerations

CHILD AND ADOLESCENT PSYCHIATRIC CLINICS

ISSUE OF RELATED INTEREST

Pediatric Clinics of North America, December 2016 (Vol. 63, No. 6)
Lesbian, Gay, Bisexual, and Transgender Youth
Stewart L. Adelson, Nadia L. Dowshen, Harvey J. Makadon, and Robert Garofalo,
Editors
Available at: http://www.pediatric.theclinics.com/

AACAP Members: Please go to www.jaacap.org for information on access to the Child and Adolescent Psychiatric Clinics. *Resident* Members of AACAP: Special access information is available at www.childpsych.theclinics.com.

THE CLINICS ARE AVAILABLE ONLINE!
Access your subscription at:
www.theclinics.com

Preface

Co-occurring Medical Illnesses in Child and Adolescent Psychiatry: Updates and Treatment Considerations

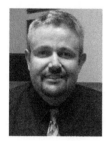

Matthew D. Willis, MD, MPH, FAAP
Editor

In our current medical era of ever-increasing subspecialization and resultantly fragmented clinical care, the need for truly integrated and collaborative clinical work has never been more pronounced. Sadly, however, given the significant time demands associated with clinical collaboration and communication across specialties and the lack of financial incentives accompanying this work, it is all too common in today's era for clinicians to find themselves operating within individual silos with little to no contact with other medical providers. Among physicians, and in particular in outpatient settings, there is perhaps nowhere in medicine where this issue is more pronounced than in psychiatry, where regular collaborative communication with other medical providers at times appears to be the exception rather than the norm.

The ultimate underlying causes for this pattern of "siloed" care are probably multifactorial and complex, but among these factors appears to be a pattern of psychiatrists "losing touch" with their medical training over time as well as losing academic and clinical interest in physical conditions and diagnoses outside of their specialized realm of patient care. As this occurs, what is notably also lost by way of this process is an appreciation for the ways in which physical conditions profoundly impact emotional health as well as an appreciation for how a broad and up-to-date medical knowledge base is essential for optimal and effective psychiatric treatment.

This need for psychiatrists to maintain a solid and wide-ranging multidisciplinary knowledge base is perhaps most critical in child and adolescent psychiatry, where psychoeducation and other treatment modalities are focused not only on the patient but also on the family. Consider, for example, the depressed adolescent whose

Child Adolesc Psychiatric Clin N Am 27 (2018) xi–xii
https://doi.org/10.1016/j.chc.2017.10.001
1056-4993/18/© 2017 Published by Elsevier Inc.

childpsych.theclinics.com

parents are worried about "chronic Lyme disease," the anxious child who has developed seizurelike episodes in the context of recent reexposure to historically traumatic stimuli, or the previously overweight teenager who is now bradycardic and orthostatic after rapidly "successful" weight loss. In each of these clinical scenarios, effective psychoeducation and subsequent treatment depend upon a solid medical knowledge base outside of the field of psychiatry. This critical knowledge base, for example, helps the practicing child and adolescent psychiatrist to distinguish structural from emotional causes (eg, Lyme disease vs major depressive disorder, epileptic vs nonepileptic seizures), and to help patients and families to identify the clinical "red flags" that distinguish health-promoting and medically dangerous behaviors (eg, "healthy" lifestyle changes vs an emerging eating disorder).

It was with this essential working knowledge base in mind that this issue of the *Child and Adolescent Psychiatric Clinics of North America* was conceptualized, and high yield multidisciplinary topics relevant to the practice of child and adolescent psychiatry were chosen. We are greatly indebted to the esteemed authors from across the various pediatric specialties who accepted our challenge to provide concise yet detailed reviews of these topics and to structure these articles in a way that is both academically rigorous yet applicable to everyday clinical practice. It is our hope that this issue will offer practicing child and adolescent psychiatrists increased interest in these high-yield topics, increased proactivity in communicating and collaborating with other medical providers with whom they share patients, and increased confidence in their ability to care for their most complicated patients.

Matthew D. Willis, MD, MPH, FAAP
Hasbro Children's Partial Hospital Program
Department of Psychiatry and Human Behavior
The Alpert Medical School of Brown University
Rhode Island Hospital
Potter Building
593 Eddy Street
Providence, RI 02903

E-mail address:
MWillis1@Lifespan.org

Medical Considerations in Children and Adolescents with Eating Disorders

Diane DerMarderosian, MD[a],*, Heather A. Chapman, MD[a],
Christina Tortolani, PhD[b], Matthew D. Willis, MD, MPH[c]

KEYWORDS

- Eating disorders • Bradycardia • Orthostasis • Malnutrition • Abnormal weight loss
- Restriction • Refeeding • Integrated care

KEY POINTS

- Eating disorders are psychiatric disorders with significant, potentially fatal, medical complications. Appropriate screening and assessment facilitate timely, intensive, integrated care essential to optimizing outcomes.
- The first priorities in treatment should include nutritional rehabilitation, weight restoration, and medical stability; this supports optimal engagement in psychological treatment required for full recovery.
- Refeeding syndrome represents the metabolic and clinical changes that occur when a malnourished patient is not judiciously renourished and can result in cardiovascular collapse and potential death.
- Family-based treatment has been found to be most effective in supporting longer term remission for children and adolescents with eating disorders.
- The best outcomes for children and adolescents with eating disorders are associated with a collaborative approach and shared decision making among an interdisciplinary team and family.

Disclosures: The authors have no disclosures.
[a] Department of Pediatrics, Hasbro Children's Partial Hospital Program, Alpert Medical School at Brown University, 593 Eddy Street, Providence, RI 02903, USA; [b] Department of Counseling, Educational Leadership and School Psychology, Rhode Island College, Alpert Medical School at Brown University, 600 Mount Pleasant Avenue, Providence, RI 02908, USA; [c] Department of Psychiatry and Human Behavior, Hasbro Children's Partial Hospital Program, Alpert Medical School at Brown University, 593 Eddy Street, Providence, RI 02903, USA
* Corresponding author. Hasbro Children's Partial Hospital Program, Potter Basement 593 Eddy Street, Providence, RI 02903, USA.
E-mail address: DDerMarderosian@Lifespan.org

Child Adolesc Psychiatric Clin N Am 27 (2018) 1–14
http://dx.doi.org/10.1016/j.chc.2017.08.002
1056-4993/18/© 2017 Elsevier Inc. All rights reserved.

childpsych.theclinics.com

```
Abbreviations
BMI   Body mass index
EKG   Electrocardiograph
FBT   Family-based treatment
HR    Heart rate
```

INTRODUCTION

Eating disorders are a group of psychiatric illnesses with significant, potentially fatal, medical complications requiring early detection and treatment for optimal outcome.[1] Included in the *Diagnostic and Statistical Manual of Mental Disorders,* 5th edition, Feeding and Eating Disorder classification are anorexia nervosa, bulimia nervosa, binge eating disorder, and "other" and "unspecified" categories, all of which include elements of body image distortion and are referred to in this article collectively as "eating disorders." Acknowledging that diagnosis is the first step to treatment, it is important to understand that patients with limited weight loss, or seemingly brief duration of illness, can be at risk for medical complications and negative outcomes necessitating medical assessment and treatment.[1] It is critical to involve clinicians familiar with these issues and open to interdisciplinary collaboration, which includes primary medical providers, therapists, psychiatrists, dieticians, and family.[2]

Early, intensive, integrated treatment for patients with eating disorders and their families is associated with improved prognosis and outcomes. Moreover, a delay in appropriate treatment is associated with medical, psychological, and social complications, which may not be reversible.[3] Many potentially life-threatening medical sequelae are difficult to detect or are nondetectable with medical testing, and patients who die from medical complications of their illness often have normal laboratory test values. Of note, suicide attempts and completed suicides are relatively common, especially for patients with bingeing and/or purging behaviors, and a diagnosis of anorexia nervosa is associated with the highest mortality rate of any psychiatric disorder.[2]

Owing to the complexity of these illnesses, the lack of clear markers for severity or risk, and potential negative outcomes, a comprehensive understanding of all eating disorder symptoms (thoughts, behaviors, and medical information) is critical for appropriately assessing medical needs, level of risk, and required interventions. Because early diagnosis and multidisciplinary treatment result in better outcomes, it is crucial to solicit and recognize unhealthy thoughts, behaviors, and patterns related to food, body, and health that require treatment, even if an individual denies such thoughts or minimizes their significance.[2] Primary medical and psychological providers play a key role in early detection of eating disorders. Routine screening is essential and should be performed in the context of all preteen and adolescent annual health supervision and sports clearance visits. As recommended by the American Academy of Child and Adolescent Psychiatry, all preteen and adolescent patients, regardless of the reason for presentation, should be asked about eating patterns and body satisfaction.[4]

DIAGNOSIS
Screening

It is important for providers to screen routinely for eating disorders and to identify signs and symptoms suggestive of disordered eating. Routine monitoring should include of height, weight and body mass index (BMI) longitudinally on growth charts to identify concerning trends, even if weight loss is absent or an individual seems at a healthy weight or overweight.[5] The Bright Futures guidelines and/or the SCOFF questionnaire can provide a helpful framework to screen for concerning thoughts and behaviors. If warranted, further assessment can occur in the primary medical setting, or by referring to appropriate subspecialists. This assessment should include evaluating medical and nutritional status including level of psychiatric safety.[2]

The differential diagnosis (**Box 1**) is extensive and should be explored thoroughly to diagnose and treat the patient appropriately. This includes consideration of comorbid medical and/or psychiatric diagnoses. Key medical populations to consider are those with type 1 diabetes mellitus, thyroid disease, and inflammatory bowel disease.[6]

Evaluation (History, Review of Systems, Examination, Laboratory Studies)

Obtaining a collateral history from parents or other support people is imperative, because individuals with eating disorders have impaired perceptions of health, body, and food. Medical and nutritional history, physical examination, and selected laboratory tests are performed to clarify the diagnosis, determine severity, and guide treatment. A comprehensive history includes questions about past highest and lowest weight, desired weight, perceived healthy weight, and exercise history, including how the patient feels on days she or he cannot exercise. In addition, a dietary history including daily intake, portion sizes, food restrictions, picky eating, ritualized eating habits, calorie/fat/carbohydrate counting, and amounts of noncaloric fluid intake is essential. Exploring bingeing and purging history (including vomiting, laxative use, diuretic use, ipecac use, and overexercise), anabolic steroid use, stimulant or other drug use, menstrual history, elimination history, and physical/sexual abuse history is necessary. A family history should also be obtained and should include questions about obesity, eating disorders, depression, other mental illness, and substance abuse.[2]

A complete review of systems should be obtained to determine the presence of symptoms associated with malnutrition, purging or other medical causes of weight loss. Pertinent positives on review of systems are found in **Box 2**. Physical

---

Box 1
Differential diagnosis of eating disorders

Endocrine
   Hypothyroidism, diabetes mellitus, other endocrine disorders (hypopituitarism, Addison disease)

Gastrointestinal
   Inflammatory bowel disease
   Celiac disease

Infectious disease
   Chronic infections (human immunodeficiency virus, tuberculosis, others)

Other psychological disorders
   Obsessive–compulsive disorder
   Anxiety disorders
   Depression
   Substance abuse

Other disorders
   Central nervous system lesions (including malignancies)
   Other cancers
   Superior mesenteric artery syndrome

Box 2
Symptoms (pertinent positives) found in patients with eating disorders

Anorexia nervosa
  Amenorrhea
  Infertility
  Irritability
  Depression
  Exertional fatigue
  Weakness
  Headache
  Dizziness
  Chest pain
  Faintness
  Constipation
  Nonfocal abdominal pain
  Feeling of "fullness" with eating
  Polyuria
  Dry skin
  Intolerance of cold
  Low back pain

Bulimia nervosa
  Irregular menses
  Heart palpitations
  Esophageal burning
  Lethargy
  Fatigue
  Headache
  Constipation/diarrhea
  Swelling of hands/feet
  Frequent sore throat
  Depression
  Swollen cheeks

From Mehler P, Andersen AE. Eating disorders: a guide to medical care and complications. 2nd edition. Baltimore (MD): Johns Hopkins Press; 2010; with permission.

---

examination findings found in patients with eating disorders are numerous (**Box 3**). A full screening should be performed with the understanding that normal laboratory values do not exclude medical instability or serious illness. Initial assessment includes a complete blood count, a compete metabolic panel, liver function tests, urinalysis, thyroid function tests, erythrocyte sedimentation rate, total IgA, and tissue transglutaminase. An electrocardiograph (EKG) should also be completed looking for abnormalities including altered heart rate (HR), voltage, and repolarization. In patients with amenorrhea, a pregnancy test, luteinizing hormone, follicle-stimulating hormone, estradiol, and prolactin should be performed. Other testing including imaging (computed tomography, MRI, upper and lower gastrointestinal system studies) should be performed if clinically indicated. In boys, a free and total testosterone is done. A bone density study is recommended in girls with amenorrhea for more than 6 months or in boys with severe malnutrition, acute weight loss, or low testosterone. Low levels of testosterone can be associated with nutritional compromise.[1]

Complications

Eating disorders can affect every organ system. Children and adolescents are at particular risk owing to their active phase of growth and development. Medical

---

Box 3
Physical signs found in individuals with eating disorders

Anorexia nervosa
  Cachexia
  Hypothermia
  Bradycardia (heart rate <60 bpm)
  Hypotension
  Orthostatic vital sign changes
  Hypoactive bowel sounds
  Dry skin
  Pressure sores
  Brittle hair
  Brittle nails
  Hair loss on scalp
  "Yellow" skin, especially palms
  Lanugo hair
  Cyanotic and cold hands and feet
  Edema (ankle, periorbital)
  Heart murmur (mitral valve prolapse)

Bulimia nervosa
  Calluses on the back of the hand (Russell's sign)
  Salivary glad hypertrophy (swollen cheeks)
  Erosion of dental enamel (perimolysis)
  Periodontal disease
  Dental caries
  Facial petechiae
  Perioral irritation
  Mouth ulcer
  Hematemesis (vomiting blood)
  Edema (ankle, periorbital)
  Abdominal bloating
  Cardiac arrhythmia

From Mehler P, Andersen AE. Eating disorders: a guide to medical care and complications. 2nd edition. Baltimore (MD): Johns Hopkins Press; 2010; with permission.

---

complications associated with eating disorders can be caused by malnutrition, bingeing/purging behaviors, or refeeding. If medical complications are identified, they should be addressed immediately.[1] The majority of medical complications resolve after judicious nutritional restoration, resolution of unhealthy eating behaviors, and recovery from the eating disorder. However, potentially irreversible medical effects include growth retardation, loss of dental enamel in the context of chronic vomiting, structural brain changes, pubertal delay/arrest, and impaired acquisition of peak bone mass and subsequent increase in fracture risk.[3]

Treatment

As stated, early, integrated care is critical in the treatment of patients with eating disorders to improve prognosis and minimize morbidity and mortality. As part of the initial evaluation, it is important to determine the most appropriate level of care, which can include inpatient medical, inpatient psychiatric, residential, or partial and intensive outpatient treatment, although resources vary based on location. If significant medical or nutritional compromise exists, an inpatient medical stay may be necessary. The Society for Adolescent Medicine recommends inpatient admission if 1 or more of the following is present: severe malnutrition (weight <75% ideal body weight), dehydration, electrolyte disturbance, cardiac dysrhythmia, physiologic instability (bradycardia with HR <50 daytime and <45 at night), hypotension (80/50 mm Hg), orthostatic changes in HR, arrested growth and development, failure of outpatient treatment, uncontrollable bingeing and purging, acute medical complications of malnutrition, acute psychiatric emergencies, or comorbid diagnoses that interfere with treatment.[3]

If an inpatient medical admission is required for stabilization, judicious refeeding is essential. This includes slow, progressive advancement of balanced nutrition, including appropriate percentages of carbohydrate, protein, and fat.[7] Patients require close monitoring through this process for evidence of refeeding syndrome—metabolic disturbances that occur as a result of reinstitution of nutrition to malnourished patients. This monitoring includes frequent laboratory testing, because the refeeding process can precipitate significant abnormalities that require immediate treatment.

Refeeding syndrome is defined as severe electrolyte and fluid shifts that occur in the early stages of rapid and injudicious nutritional replenishment. In the starved state, metabolism shifts to catabolism, breaking down tissue including fat and muscle to access the energy required to maintain essential bodily functions. With refeeding, metabolism returns to anabolism, a state of body building and repair. This process requires increased uptake of electrolytes including potassium, phosphate, and magnesium. A sudden change in the concentrations of these electrolytes can stress the heart, causing serious complications including arrhythmias. Refeeding syndrome can affect almost every body system leading to respiratory, cardiac, neurologic, gastrointestinal, and skeletal problems.[8]

Regardless of the level of care, early, multidisciplinary treatment including nutritional, medical, and mental health professionals is a cornerstone of successful treatment. For psychological interventions to be effective, medical stabilization and nutritional rehabilitation are imperative. There is growing evidence that individual based therapies, such as interpersonal psychotherapy, enhanced cognitive therapy, dialectical behavior therapy, and acceptance and commitment therapy can positively impact short-term outcomes. However, family-based treatment (FBT) has been found to be the most effective in supporting longer term remission for children and adolescents who have been ill for less than 3 years, are under the age of 18, and are medically stable for outpatient treatment.[9,10]

FBT encompasses 3 phases of treatment over 6 to 12 months with an emphasis on parental symptom management. The family's role shifts depending on the phase. During phase I, family members mobilize to take charge of their child's eating (and related behaviors), much like an inpatient staff would. During later phases, as the adolescent restores weight and becomes less immersed in the eating disorder pathology, he or she is gradually given back control over eating. Throughout the treatment, care givers support parents to "fight the eating disorder" with a "food as medicine" approach. By getting the adolescent "back on track" and returned to normal development, care givers and parents treat the eating disorder and prevent relapses. Although FBT was developed for an outpatient setting, its principles have begun to be adapted for use across levels of care, including inpatient, partial hospitalization, and intensive outpatient treatment.[10–12]

Psychopharmacology often plays a key role in this patient population. Comorbid anxiety disorders and depressive disorders are common in patients with eating disorders, and these potential comorbidities often drive the selection of psychiatric medications. Notably, research demonstrates that weight restoration in itself improves obsessive thought processes, compulsive behaviors, and mood lability. Thus, in the absence of clearly identified comorbid psychiatric disorders, nutritional repletion should be considered the first line treatment for eating disorder–associated anxiety and/or mood disturbance. Psychiatric medications should be considered, however, when comorbid psychiatric diagnoses are identified, when mood or anxiety symptoms persist with ongoing nutritional repletion, or when anxiety symptoms are so severe that they pose significant challenges with regard to initial eating disorder treatment adherence.

In the clinical situations noted, psychiatric medications of potential therapeutic value include selective serotonin reuptake inhibitors, benzodiazepines, and atypical antipsychotics. Of note, there are no US Food and Drug Administration (FDA)–approved medications for the treatment of eating disorders in adolescents, and only fluoxetine possesses FDA approval for bulimia nervosa in adults. As such, all of the recommended approaches delineated herein are off label, but potentially valuable. With regard to selective serotonin reuptake inhibitors, given that eating disorders share similar clinical features with obsessive–compulsive disorder (highly ruminative thought processes and obsessive behaviors around nutrition, body image, and exercise), and given that both medicines are approved by the FDA for the treatment of pediatric obsessive–compulsive disorder, we recommend that sertraline or fluoxetine be considered when functional impairment related to these symptoms is significant. Despite also sharing FDA approval for pediatric obsessive–compulsive disorder, clomipramine should be avoided in this patient population, related to potential cardiac side effects in patients already at risk for cardiac abnormalities. Additionally, our own anecdotal experience is that fluvoxamine (also approved for pediatric obsessive–compulsive disorder) has limited value given daytime sedation as a common side effect. Escitalopram can also be considered (particularly if family history indicates a therapeutic response in a relative) given FDA approval and reasonably efficacy data for this medication in pediatric major depressive disorder (often comorbid with eating disorders). Citalopram should not be considered first line in this population owing to statistical association with electrolyte abnormalities and QT prolongation. In addition, bupropion should be avoided, given the potential for cardiac abnormalities, seizures, and weight loss.

Benzodiazepines should be considered when premeal and/or postmeal anxiety poses significant challenges with regard to nutritional adherence. In such situations, lorazepam is commonly chosen owing to its intermediate pharmacokinetics (providing immediate benefit if given 30 minutes before a meal while also typically remaining therapeutically active for snacks scheduled between meal times). If given, a standing 3 times daily schedule is recommended, typically for a period of several weeks while selective serotonin reuptake inhibitors are concomitantly titrated to effect. Our own experience is that as-needed use of benzodiazepines is often complicated by patients' difficulties identifying their own distress despite clear outward evidence thereof, or owing to ambivalence about taking medication that may facilitate improved nutritional adherence.

Although not considered as first line as the recommendations provided, atypical antipsychotics can have therapeutic value in patients with eating disorders, particularly when distorted and/or ruminative cognitions around body image and nutritional content border on being delusional in quality or severity. In these situations, we most commonly consider olanzapine, given several studies demonstrating modest therapeutic value in patients with restrictive eating disorders,[13,14] typical immediate therapeutic efficacy if patients respond favorably, and anecdotal experience that olanzapine's side effect profile (appetite stimulation and sedation in particular) is often advantageous in this patient population. Of note, mild sedation is often welcomed in patients and families given the degree of agitation that can be associated with meal times, and this sedation can typically be minimized while preserving therapeutic efficacy by way of evening dosing.

Despite their relative prevalence, misconceptions persist among professionals and the public regarding the medical and psychological risks associated with eating disorders. The following case provide an opportunity to highlight common areas of misunderstanding and provide education.

CASE

AB is a 15-year-old natal and self-identified female with restrictive eating, excessive exercise, weight loss, and amenorrhea referred to the eating disorder medical team for treatment of a presumed eating disorder. Record review showed an 18 month history of weight loss in the context of height growth. Her BMI was initially 23, decreasing in that time to 19.1. About 1.5 years ago, AB decided to "get healthy" through dietary changes and increased exercise.

Her parents described her as previously unconcerned with food, eating "more than she needed to at times" and "a little on the pudgy side." They reported that she initially began cutting out "junk food," "carbs," and sugary beverages while increasing lean proteins, fruits, vegetables, and water intake. At the same time, she began running 6 to 7 times per week. In the first few months of these behavioral changes, AB and her family perceived this as a good change, and she received positive feedback from peers, family, and her medical providers about her appearance and apparent healthy decisions.

Six months ago, AB's parents became concerned about continued weight loss, irritability in food discussions, excessive exercise, and rigidity around food intake (cutting out all desserts and sweets, avoiding fats like salad dressing and butter). Additional unhealthy behaviors included evidence of viewing Pro-Ana websites, spending excessive amounts of time meal planning, preparing food for others that she would not eat herself, and not allowing anyone else to prepare food for her. At this time, her parents were allowing AB to be "in charge of her own food, because at least she will eat something this way." As a result of their concerns, her parents spoke with her pediatrician, who reassured the family that the patient's BMI was normal, and that there was no reason to be concerned.

According to AB, she started making changes to her diet starting 1.5 years ago after "getting sick of people making fun of how much I ate and my weight." She identified restriction and exercise as the main components of her weight loss efforts. Over the past few months, she had realized that eating had taken control of her life, and she expressed concern about the impact on her health and lifestyle. However, AB's fear of weight gain was so severe that she had been unsuccessful in making changes. On questioning, AB reported thinking about food, weight, and shape upwards of 90% of her day. She denied a history of bingeing, purging, or use of laxatives, diuretics, or diet pills.

Eating and exercise history revealed that AB had increased water and green tea intake considerably, and chewed approximately 1 pack of gum per day. Her exercise pattern included running 5 miles, 6 days a week as well as playing in the school soccer league daily. Family and patient agree on her daily intake:

- Breakfast: oatmeal made with water, apple, green tea, water
- Lunch: packs Greek yogurt, apple, raw broccoli, strawberries, water
- Dinner: prepares separate meal from parents, chicken or fish, salad with no dressing, steamed vegetables, water
- After school snack: almonds, grapes

Her family history is notable for untreated anxiety in her mother and maternal grandmother. Mother reports, "I have always had to watch my weight. I pay a lot of attention to what I am eating and if I eat too much, I tend to focus on exercising." There was no indication of further family psychiatric illness and no history of diagnosed eating disorders. Social history reveals that AB lives at home with her parents and siblings (13-year-old brother and 18-year-old sister). There was no history of trauma, violence in the home, or physical, sexual, or verbal abuse. There was no known history of Department of Youth and Family Services involvement, and no indication of substance use. AB is a sophomore at her local public high school where she receives As in honors classes. She has distanced herself from her friends who seem frustrated with her eating behaviors. There is no report or indication of substance use.

AB was referred to a pediatrician who specialized in eating disorders for further evaluation. Her pertinent medical history includes amenorrhea with her last menstrual period 4 months ago; before this, menses were irregular and "light" for the previous 6 months. She reported feeling dizzy and lightheaded with standing. Her sitting HR on physical examination was 62 bpm. Routine evaluation included orthostatic vital signs, which demonstrated orthostasis by HR (55–95 bpm) and systolic blood pressure (99/58–85/50). An EKG was ordered and demonstrated critical bradycardia with a HR of 44 bpm. Additional relevant medical findings included acrocyanosis, cool hands and feet, and was otherwise normal. Laboratory testing revealed low zinc and prealbumin. All other laboratory tests, including albumin, were normal.

Based on her bradycardia in the context of acute weight loss and entrenched eating disorder cognitions and behaviors, inpatient medical admission was indicated. Early in her inpatient stay, AB's overnight HR nadir was 32 bpm. Over the course of her admission, as she was judiciously refed, AB stabilized medically as reflected by resolution of her orthostasis and bradycardia. Laboratory tests were monitored regularly for evidence of refeeding syndrome. She shifted from a hypometabolic state evidenced by her bradycardia, orthostasis, low temperature, and acrocyanosis, to a hypermetabolic state with a normal body temperature, no orthostasis, and blood pressure readings and HRs in normal range. In this state of hypermetabolism AB required a high level of nutrition to support physiologic recovery. Her nutritional needs for recovery were established during the course of her stay. After discharge, she was monitored closely by a multidisciplinary team, including a pediatrician, therapist, psychiatrist, and dietician, all of whom communicated regularly around her care.

CLINICAL PEARLS
Pearl #1

"Her BMI is normal. There is nothing to worry about."

BMI, a ratio using height and weight, is a deceiving measure. It does not take into account body composition, and is not a categorical measure of an individual's overall health. BMI is a population screening tool that offers a quantitative measure of how an individual's weight-to-height compares with others. BMI does not differentiate between fat and muscle mass, so athletes will often have BMIs deemed "overweight." It tells nothing about the actual health of the person it is measuring and provides no temporal context (recent weight decreases, increases, etc). It is especially difficult to use BMI to evaluate children as they go through growth spurts or may be growth delayed from illness. Moreover, the active period of growth and development during preadolescence and adolescence place them at risk for significant compromise in this context.

Determining a goal treatment weight can be a complex process. A healthy weight supports the normal physiology of adolescence, including puberty, growth and development, physical activity, and improved psychological functioning. Weight restoration is associated with resumption of spontaneous menses, which leads to improved bone mineral density. Considerations include premorbid trajectory for height, weight, and BMI, age at pubertal onset, and current pubertal stage. During a period of growth, the individual's treatment goal weight should be reassessed every 3 to 6 months.[3] Goal treatment weight during childhood and adolescence is often a moving target, taking into account natural growth and physical development that occurs during these critical years is essential. As evidenced on the growth curves published by the Centers for Disease Control and Prevention, the goal treatment weight for a 13-year-old is not ideal for a 17-year-old, even at the same height.[2]

A full recovery profile (rather than alleviation of 1 symptom) includes sustained weight restoration without continued engagement in eating disordered behaviors, flexible cognitions around food intake, and return of bodily functions and to growth curve. Many patients need to weigh more than they ever did before to resume their menses, possibly related to past menses being anovulatory. Other reasons why target weight restoration goals often exceed any past weights for a given child include a history of stunted growth and development in the context of undernutrition, the corresponding need for "catch-up" growth to address this, and increased metabolic needs related to pubertal growth and development until the body finds its "set point."[15]

Many people with eating disorders do not seem to be sick. It is impossible to tell whether a person is underweight by appearance alone. Because ideal body weights are highly individualized based on bone structure, muscle mass, body shape, and weight history, a person may fall within the "ideal" BMI range and still be significantly malnourished. If these patients are not properly evaluated, they may be missed and may not receive timely, necessary treatment.

Pearl #2

"She is eating 3 meals and snacks every day. Her eating is not a problem."

A comprehensive nutritional assessment and sophisticated understanding of the medical implications of compromised nutritional status is essential. Eating meals and snacks alone does not make an appropriate diet. Exploring details about specific content of intake as well as level activity is critical. Consideration of energy balance between dietary energy intake and energy expenditure required for health and activities of daily living, growth, and sporting activities is critical. A review of patterns of rigidity and rule-bound eating, including absolute elimination of food groups or food types (eg, fats and/or carbohydrates), is equally essential.[3]

The first steps in treatment should include nutritional rehabilitation, weight restoration, and medical stability. Research demonstrates that many of the physical and mental symptoms of eating disorders are caused or exacerbated by malnutrition, restrictive eating, and other unhealthy eating behaviors. As stated, the evidence supports the assertion that these symptoms diminish with normalized eating and weight restoration. A weight-recovered, nutritionally and medically stable patient with an eating disorder is better equipped to manage eating disorder triggers and begin psychological recovery.

Weight restoration is an essential prerequisite to full recovery. Waiting for patients to feel comfortable eating and start doing so on their own is not an effective approach. Instead, providing the support to families to feed their children despite resistance is recommended. In weight gain after semistarvation, the fat distribution begins around the face and stomach. The mechanism for this is not understood, but it does redistribute over time. Understanding this pattern and providing guidance to families is vital to facilitating ongoing caregiver adherence to a highly structured and closely supervised meal plan.[16] In the absence of this education and support, parents are at risk for succumbing to their own fears about "making my child fat" and becoming nonadherent to necessary treatment.

Pearl #3

"Wow! That is way too much food."

The body conserves energy in a state of undernutrition, and requires a significant amount of nutrition to recover. Judicious refeeding with close medical monitoring is imperative, often requiring an inpatient level of care initially to ensure medical safety. Patients have high nutritional needs throughout their recovery to "make up for lost time" and medically rehabilitate. Of note, they become very sensitive to activity, with clearance for even functional activities often requiring a nutritional increase to accommodate metabolic needs.

The conservatory response is wide reaching. Menstrual periods become irregular and stop. Breathing, pulse, and blood pressure rates drop. Thyroid function slows. At times, laboratory tests resemble euthyroid sick syndrome (low T3, low T4 and normal or low thyroid-stimulating hormone). When this picture exists in the context of malnutrition, the only recommended intervention is nutritional rehabilitation. Nails and hair become brittle. Skin gets dry, yellows, and lanugo grows. Gastrointestinal transit slows and contributes to constipation. Reduced body fat leads to lowered body temperatures.[1]

When a patient is inadequately nourished, structural, functional, and metabolic alterations can result. Injudicious nutritional therapy can lead to adverse clinical consequences known as refeeding syndrome.[7] Refeeding syndrome is defined as the metabolic and clinical changes that occur when a malnourished patient is aggressively nutritionally rehabilitated.[8] If not recognized and treated properly, refeeding syndrome can result in cardiovascular collapse and potential death that follows the refeeding of undernourished individuals with highly caloric nutrients (especially those high in glucose). Refeeding syndrome is a concern for any patient who has been without consistent or adequate nutrition for a prolonged period of time. Serious complications can be avoided with appropriate identification of patients at risk, slow initiation of feeding with appropriately balanced nutrition, and careful monitoring.[8]

Pearl #4

"Her vital signs and laboratory tests were normal in my office this afternoon. She cannot be that sick."

It is important to assess and monitor patients with eating disorders longitudinally in the medical setting as early as possible. Patients with eating disorders have the highest premature mortality rates of any diagnoses in the *Diagnostic and Statistical Manual of Mental Disorders*.[1] They are at greater risk of dying prematurely than almost any other like-aged patient admitted to the medical hospital. The medical consequences of eating disorders are broad reaching. A set of "normal" routine vital signs does not confirm medical stability. Many factors can contribute to increasing HR so that it seems to be "normal," including anxiety, anemia, dehydration, caffeine, and stimulants. It is important to properly assess vital signs to get the most accurate information possible, which includes performing orthostatic vital signs as well as an EKG. This case demonstrates that a sitting HR can be deceivingly reassuring.[17]

Cardiac considerations include bradycardia, which can be a marker of the metabolic downshift that occurs to conserve energy when there is not enough nutrition available. Of note, this is not only due to athleticism. Orthostasis, an increase in HR and/or decrease in blood pressure with positional change, can represent nutritional compromise as well. This occurs when the heart muscle (like the rest of the body) is compromised in size and function owing to inadequate nutrition. It is important to remember that low HRs do not demonstrate fitness in the context of abnormal weight loss, undernutrition/underweight, orthostasis, symptoms of dizziness and lightheadedness, or eating disordered behaviors.[17]

If the heart is unable to mount appropriate contractility to support conservation of blood pressure with positional changes, it initially compensates with increased HR with standing, which does maintain the blood pressure. Over time, if HR variability has been impacted by undernutrition, the heart is unable to increase HR and has no way to preserve the blood pressure, which manifests clinically as lightheadedness (presyncope) and fainting (syncope). Anything that decreases blood volume (dehydration), hemoglobin (anemia), or causes vasodilatation (warm showers/baths) can exacerbate this condition. A new murmur can emerge if the cardiac muscle mass decreases with resulting mitral valve prolapse. EKG findings can include a long QTc, QT dispersion, poor HR variability, low voltage, and critical arrhythmias in the context of exercise (identified on stress test).[17] Fortunately, these clinical alterations can all resolve with nutritional recovery.

There are limited "absolute" measures for understanding medical compromise and severity. People die from the complications of eating disorders with normal laboratory tests. Once there are obvious signs of medical compromise, the illness, including its medical impact, is often quite progressed. Although very low weight is a risk factor for medical severity, amount of weight lost and weight decrease from a patient's usual weight curve (weight suppression) are also associated with significant medical risk. Understanding a patient's weight trends and level of activity is essential. Of note, patients with comorbid medical issues like diabetes are at the greatest risk.[1]

Pearl #5

"She is fine from a medical point of view. Talk to her therapist about what she thinks."

To treat patients with eating disorders optimally, an interdisciplinary team of providers who actively communicate between one another is critical. The best outcomes for children and adolescents with eating disorders are associated with a collaborative approach by an interdisciplinary team, including providers trained in FBT.[9] As providers, we must talk to each other and to families. A unified message is essential. Decision making should come from an interdisciplinary perspective including the family. For example, even if a patient seems medically stable enough to be cleared for exercise, it may not be indicated owing to his or her psychological state or past triggers. Almost without exception, decisions about changes in treatment plans (meal supervision, exercise allowance, etc) should be made collectively and with confirmation of agreement between providers, and not unilaterally. Mental health providers should be consulted in the decision making around when and how to potentially liberalize meal supervision and/or exercise allowance, and should understand that their input with regard to a patient's psychological state is a critical component of this decision-making process. In fact, it is the mental health provider who is often in the lead with this collaboration with providers and communication of recommendations to the patient and family. This necessary approach requires communication between medical and psychiatric providers at each decision-making juncture. Although this might initially strike outpatient providers as excessively time intensive, it is our experience that once active lines of communication are established (often by confidential email and/or shared electronic medical records as an efficient means of correspondence), time is ultimately saved and unnecessary crises related to clinical deterioration are averted. Supporting patients and families in understanding the inextricable link between nutrition, medical status, and psychological status is imperative, and making decisions in a collaborative way further emphasizes this message.

Pearl #6

"It's my fault she has an eating disorder."

Family members of children with eating disorders often experience high levels of distress, including feelings of guilt and self-blame, which can interfere with treatment effectiveness. Through its empowering of parents to manage their child's eating disorder, and its firm, consistent, yet compassionate focus on refeeding, FBT signifies a paradigm shift in eating disorder treatment from excluding parents from treatment to holding them as the central tool for recovery. One of the main tenets of FBT is a belief that no one, including parents, is to blame for an eating disorder. FBT works to empower parents to become experts in eating disorders to "outsmart" their child's illness (disrupt all eating disordered behaviors). Parents are provided with psychoeducation, which supports them to make decisions about their child's care with a pragmatic focus on weight restoration. Parents are also encouraged to mentally separate the illness from their child and to strategize on out how to "fight" the eating disorder together.

Pearl #7

"I'm not sure that these patients ever get better."

The prognosis for children and adolescents with eating disorders in adolescents varies greatly in the literature. However, outcomes are significantly better than those reported in adults, including lower mortality rates.[18] Although the illness course is often protracted, the majority of patients recover medically, behaviorally, and psychologically from their eating disorders, especially with early intervention.

Primary providers, medical and psychological, play an invaluable role in preventing, diagnosing, and treating eating disorders. Having a high index of suspicion, being familiar with the signs and symptoms of eating disorders, and being knowledgeable of available treatments are critical for early diagnosis, which leads to improved outcomes and is potentially life saving. Moreover, longitudinal providers, based on their longstanding relationships with families, can provide vital support, because these illnesses have a significant impact on all family members.

REFERENCES

1. Golden N, Katzman D, Sawyer S, et al. Position paper of the society for adolescent health and medicine: medical management of restrictive eating disorders in adolescents and young adults. J Adolesc Health 2015;56:121–5.
2. Golden N, Katzman D, Kreipe R, et al. Eating disorders in adolescents: position paper of the society of adolescent medicine. J Adolesc Health 2003;33(6): 496–503.
3. Katzman K. Medical complications in adolescents with anorexia nervosa: a review of the literature. Int J Eat Disord 2005;37(suppl):S52–9.

4. La Via M, American Academy of Child and Adolescent Psychiatry (AACAP) Committee on Quality Issues (CQI). Practice parameter for the assessment and treatment of children and adolescents with eating disorders. J Am Acad Child Adolesc Psychiatry 2015;56:121–5.
5. Dickstein L, Froco K, Rome E, et al. Recognizing, managing medical consequences of eating disorders in primary care. Cleve Clin J Med 2014;81(4):255–63.
6. Mehler P, Andersen A. Eating disorders: a guide to medical care and complications. Baltimore: Johns Hopkins University Press; 2010.
7. Fuentebella J, Kerner J. Refeeding syndrome. Pediatr Clin North Am 2009;56(5):1201–10.
8. Pulcini C, Zettle S, Srinath A. Refeeding syndrome. Pediatr Rev 2016;37(12):516–23.
9. Lock J, Le Grange D, Agras W, et al. Randomized clinical trial comparing family-based treatment with adolescent-focused individual therapy for adolescents with anorexia nervosa. Arch Gen Psychiatry 2010;67(10):1025–32.
10. Lock J, Le Grange D. Treatment manual for anorexia nervosa: a family-based approach. 2nd edition. New York: Guilford Press; 2013.
11. Hoste RR. Incorporating family-based therapy principles into a partial hospitalization programme for adolescents with anorexia nervosa: challenges and considerations. J Fam Ther 2015;37:41–60.
12. Rockwell RE, Boutelle K, Trunko ME, et al. An innovative short-term, intensive, family-based treatment for adolescent anorexia nervosa: case series. Eur Eat Disord Rev 2011;19:362–7.
13. Bissada H, Tasca GA, Barber AM, et al. Olanzapine in the treatment of low body weight and obsessive thinking in women with anorexia nervosa: a randomized, double-blind, placebo-controlled trial. Am J Psychiatry 2008;165:1281.
14. Attia E, Kaplan AS, Walsh BT, et al. Olanzapine versus placebo for out-patients with anorexia nervosa. Psychol Med 2011;41:2177.
15. Golden N, Meyer W. Resumption of menses in anorexia nervosa. Arch Pediatr Adolesc Med 1997;151(4):16–21.
16. O'Toole J. Give food a chance: a new view on childhood eating disorders. London: Jessica Kingsley Publishers; 2015.
17. Sachs V, Harnke M, Mehler P, et al. Cardiovascular complications of anorexia nervosa: a systematic review. Int J Eat Disord 2016;49(3):238–48.
18. Steinhausen HC. Outcome of eating disorders. Child Adolesc Psychiatr Clin N Am 2009;18(1):225–42.

Functional Abdominal Pain and Related Syndromes

Michael Herzlinger, MD*, Carolina Cerezo, MD

KEYWORDS

- Functional abdominal pain • Irritable bowel syndrome
- Functional gastrointestinal disorders • Diagnosis • Treatment • Counseling
- Management

KEY POINTS

- Medical and mental health providers commonly encounter functional gastrointestinal disorders (FGIDs). Functional abdominal pain and irritable bowel syndrome are 2 particularly common and important FGIDs.
- Accurate diagnosis of FGIDs is important to ensure that an identifiable organic process is not missed and that appropriate treatment is delivered.
- Counseling and reassurance are critical to the management of these conditions; understanding the pathophysiology of FGIDs plays an important role in this process.

BACKGROUND

Abdominal pain in children is incredibly common. Estimates vary, but reports suggest a prevalence of about 15% of children worldwide.[1] Pain may occur as often as once per week in about 40% of school-aged children.[2] It can interfere with sleep and daily functioning; children miss school, and parents lose time at work. Hence, when children complain, their worried parents may bring them to medical attention. Abdominal pain is among the top 20 most common diagnoses of all outpatient medical visits.[3] It comprises 8% of all emergency room visits.[4] These visits frequently result in testing, which can be expensive and invasive. One pediatric gastroenterology practice estimated the average cost of work-up per patient presenting with likely benign abdominal pain at approximately $6000.[5] This testing is driven by the goal of timely identification of serious or acute gastrointestinal (GI) conditions such as hepatobiliary disease, pancreatic disease, inflammatory bowel disease, or acute surgical processes. When these are excluded, work-up may reveal less worrisome or nonacute conditions, such as *Helicobacter pylori*, celiac disease, acid peptic disease, gastroesophageal reflux

Disclosure Statement: Nothing to disclose.
Pediatric Gastroenterology, Warren Alpert Medical School of Brown University, Hasbro Children's Hospital, 593 Eddy Street, Providence, RI 02903, USA
* Corresponding author.
E-mail address: mherzlinger@lifespan.org

disease, or eosinophilic esophagitis. But most often, testing demonstrates no anatomic or biochemical abnormality. In the past, various terms have been used to describe this condition, including chronic abdominal pain or recurrent abdominal pain. Currently, it is most often called functional abdominal pain. Though the source of this pain is benign, it can be debilitating. Providers are challenged with a distressed child and concerned parents, but without the help of a clear biomarker to guide diagnosis and treatment.

FUNCTIONAL GASTROINTESTINAL DISEASES

Functional abdominal pain is one of many functional GI disorders (FGID).[6] The pathophysiology underlying these conditions is not fully understood. The best understanding is that they result from dysfunctional interaction between the enteric nervous system, which innervates the GI tract, and the central nervous system (CNS). This interaction is more simply referred to as the brain-gut axis. There are both psychosocial and physiologic factors contributing to this process.[7]

Unfortunately, these conditions remain poorly defined, because there are no tests to provide a definitive diagnosis. Instead, they are categorized according to their specific constellation of symptoms. In an effort toward standardization, a worldwide group of experts, The Rome Working Group, has defined these terms. Their most recent publication constitutes the Rome IV criteria for FGIDs.[6] Much like the Diagnostic and Statistical Manual of Mental Disorders V (DSM V) in psychiatry, the Rome IV criteria provide clinicians with a framework upon which to diagnose and treat these commonly encountered GI conditions.

According to the Rome IV criteria, functional abdominal pain occurs at least 4 times per month, episodically or continuously, not only during physiologic events such as stooling or eating. It is distinguished from irritable bowel syndrome (IBS), which is characterized by pain associated with a change in the frequency and form of stool. It is also distinguished from functional dyspepsia, in which the pain or burning occurs in the upper abdomen, specifically related to eating (postprandial fullness and early satiety). The pain associated with abdominal migraine is described as paroxysmal, severe, and associated with nausea, vomiting, anorexia, photophobia, or headache. Episodes are stereotypical, discrete, and separated by weeks to months, with symptom-free periods in between bouts. The term functional abdominal pain not otherwise specified was recently updated in order to distinguish it from the pain associated with these other FGIDs[8](Table 1). Defining these terms is critical for researchers to ensure appropriate characterization of study populations. Adherence to Rome criteria allows uniformity of subject groups, ensuring comparisons are apples to apples.

A familiarity with these terms is also helpful in clinical care. However, in a busy practice, the Rome criteria can be cumbersome, so they are not strictly used. Patients may overlap multiple syndromes or may not fully meet criteria. Nevertheless, they are critical to the understanding of these conditions as positive diagnoses. Much like a migraine headache, functional abdominal pain is real and at times debilitating. Like headaches, FGIDs lack a simple blood test, although this does not prevent clinicians from providing an unequivocal diagnosis and a clear treatment plan. This is in contrast to past frameworks, which conceptualized FGIDs as negative diagnoses. In this scenario, the focus was on excluding identifiable organic sources of abdominal pain first. When testing returned unrevealing, patients were told, everything is normal; yet they remained symptomatic. This contradiction resulted in patient frustration and distrust toward the provider. When inappropriately counseled by their providers, patients heard, "it's all in your head." By conceptualizing these conditions as positive instead of negative diagnoses, therapeutic rapport is easier established, and treatment can begin.

PATHOPHYSIOLOGY UNDERLYING FUNCTIONAL GASTROINTESTINAL DISEASES

Counseling and reassurance are vital to the management of FIGDs. To do so effectively requires an understanding of the pathophysiology underlying FGIDs. Several factors contribute. Social and emotional factors play a primary role. Patients often have an intuitive understanding of this connection. It is common even for those without FGIDs to experience GI distress such as nausea, vomiting, or diarrhea just prior to a stressful event (eg, an important game for an athlete, or a high-stakes test for a student). Even more so among those with FGIDs, emotional turbulence can trigger symptoms. The overlap between emotional and GI well-being supports the notion of the brain-gut axis as a critical component underlying the pathophysiology of FGIDs.

Not only can emotional well-being influence GI symptoms, but perhaps gut factors such as the microbiome can influence the brain. Thus, it is thought that the brain-gut axis is bidirectional. Intriguing evidence to support this notion comes from mouse studies, which show differences in the behavior of antibiotic-treated mice compared with control mice.[9] Although this finding is more difficult to demonstrate in people, there may be an analogy. In another study, a group of healthy women drank a probiotic-containing fermented milk product for 4 weeks. Using functional MRI, brain activity was measured at the onset and end of the study period. This imaging detected differences in brain regions associated with emotion and sensation in the group exposed to probiotic compared with control groups.[10] Alterations in the microbiome may be implicated in FGIDs, and in IBS in particular. Although no unique IBS microbiome signature has emerged, differences in species diversity and species composition in IBS patients compared with controls have been observed.[11] These changes may account for the symptoms observed in IBS. For example, mouse studies show manipulation of the microbiome via probiotic or antibiotic administration can alter visceral sensitivity and intestinal motility.[12,13] More research is needed to clarify the mechanism by which the microbiome interacts with the gut-brain axis, resulting in GI symptoms.

Studies suggest this interaction might be mediated through the immune system.[14] Indeed there is evidence to suggest that FGIDs, IBS in particular, represent a low-grade inflammatory state. Studies have demonstrated differences in the serum cytokine, T-cell and B-cell profiles of IBS patients compared with controls.[7] Likewise, studies demonstrate mast cell hyperplasia in the small and large bowel biopsies of IBS patients compared with controls.[15] On electron microscopy, these mast cells appear in higher density surrounding enteric nerves in IBS patients compared with controls. Perhaps when mast cell products such as tryptase, histamine, and prostaglandin E−2 are released, they excite enteric sensory nerves, resulting in the symptoms associated with IBS.[16] The mechanism by which the immune system may become involved in IBS is unclear. Psychosocial stressors exacerbate inflammation in Crohn disease and ulcerative colitis.[17] They may also account for the immune system's participation in IBS.

Serotonin dysregulation also likely plays a role, with 95% of serotonin synthesized and stored in the gut, compared with only 5% in the CNS.[18] Serotonin alters intestinal motor function. Dysregulation may result in increased motility, causing diarrhea, or delayed motility, causing constipation. Serotonin is also involved in sensory

Table 1
Rome IV criteria diagnostic criteria

Functional Dyspepsia	Irritable Bowel Syndrome	Abdominal Migraine	Functional Abdominal Pain Not Otherwise Specified
Must include 1 or more of the following bothersome symptoms at least 4 d per month:	Must include all of the following:	Must include all of the following occurring at least twice:	Must be fulfilled at least 4 times per month and include all of the following:
1. Postprandial fullness	1. Abdominal pain at least 4 d per month associated with 1 or more of the following:	1. Paroxysmal episodes of intense, acute periumbilical, midline or diffuse abdominal pain lasting 1 h or more (should be the most severe and distressing symptom)	1. Episodic or continuous abdominal pain that does not occur solely during physiologic events (eg,; eating, menses)
2. Early satiation	a. Related to defecation		
3. Epigastric pain or burning not associated with defecation	b. A change in frequency of stool	2. Episodes are separated by weeks to months	2. Insufficient criteria for irritable bowel syndrome, functional dyspepsia, or abdominal migraine
4. After appropriate evaluation, the symptoms cannot be fully explained by another medical condition	c. A change in form (appearance) of stool	3. The pain is incapacitating and interferes with normal activities	
	2. In children with constipation, the pain does not resolve with resolution of the constipation (children in whom the pain resolves have functional constipation, not irritable bowel syndrome)	4. Stereotypical pattern and symptoms in the individual patient	3. After appropriate evaluation, the abdominal pain cannot be fully explained by another medical condition
Criteria fulfilled for at least 2 mo before diagnosi.		5. The pain is associated with 2 or more of the following:	Criteria fulfilled for at least 2 mo before diagnosis.
Within FD, the following subtypes are now adopted:	3. After appropriate evaluation, the symptoms cannot be fully explained by another medical condition	a. Anorexia	
1. Postprandial distress syndrome includes bothersome postprandial fullness or early satiation that prevents finishing a regular meal. Supportive features: upper abdominal bloating, postprandial nausea, or excessive belching	Criteria fulfilled for at least 2 mo before diagnosis	b. Nausea	
		c. Vomiting	
		d. Headache	
		e. Photophobia	
		f. Pallor	

2. Epigastric pain syndrome, which includes all of the following: bothersome (severe enough to interfere with normal activities) pain or burning localized to the epigastrium
   The pain is not generalized or localized to other abdominal or chest regions and is not relieved by defecation or passage of flatus Supportive criteria: (a) burning quality of the pain but without a retrosternal component and (b) pain commonly induced or relieved by ingestion of a meal but may occur while fasting

6. After appropriate evaluation, the symptoms cannot be fully explained by another medical condition.
   Criteria fulfilled for at least 6 mo before diagnosis

function; dysregulation can result in pain or nausea.[18] Sensory nerves of the intestines have plasticity. They gain efficiency in communicating pain signals to the CNS when noxious stimuli occur.[19] As a result, pain begets more pain. Any inflammatory process can initiate this cycle. The prevalence of IBS is significantly higher in those with quiescent inflammatory bowel disease and celiac disease compared with the general population.[20,21] Even infectious diarrhea can predispose to FGIDs. This concept was well demonstrated in a population study in Walkerton, Canada, after the town's reservoir was contaminated resulting in widespread serious GI infections. Eight years later, young adults who were children at the time of the outbreak were studied. Children with gastroenteritis at the time of the outbreak were found to have higher rates of IBS compared with children without infection.[22]

Although psychosocial and mental health factors may be most important, many studies suggest a biologic underpinning to FGIDs. Additional work is required to further clarify. An increased understanding of the nature of these conditions will help clinicians in diagnosis and management. In addition, when shared with patients and families, this evolving understanding of the biologic factors potentially underlying FGIDs can play a critical role in validating these conditions as positive diagnoses with real physical symptoms. These symptoms are often triggered or in some way potentiated by underlying emotional distress, but they are not fabricated. In turn, such an understanding can go a long way in destigmatizing the traditionally psychiatric interventions to which FGIDs may respond.

DIAGNOSIS

FGIDs are a positive diagnosis, not a diagnosis of exclusion; testing is not necessarily required. Much like a brain MRI is not required for all headaches, a colonoscopy is not required for all abdominal pain. Instead, obtaining a careful personal and family history, reviewing the growth chart, and performing a thorough physical examination, are usually sufficient investigation. If these are all reassuring and consistent with an FGID, one can feel confident of a correct diagnosis. On the other hand, nonreassuring findings may prompt additional work-up. Such alarm signs in the history include vomiting (especially when it is forceful, as opposed to passive regurgitation); hematemesis; chronic, severe diarrhea; pain that is focal and located outside the periumbilical region; unexplained fevers; weight loss; or impaired linear growth. A family history of inflammatory bowel disease, celiac disease, or autoimmune disease raises concern for an identifiable organic process. On physical examination, pain localizing to a particular quadrant is more worrisome than poorly localized or periumbilical pain, which is more frequently seen in functional abdominal pain. For example, right upper quadrant tenderness and hepatosplenomegaly may indicate hepatobiliary disease. Right lower quadrant pain might indicate appendicitis or ileitis of Crohn disease. Epigastric pain suggests the possibility of acid peptic disease or pancreatitis. A perianal inspection may reveal signs of Crohn disease, such as inflamed skin tags, deep fissuring, or fistulous openings.

Even in the absence of alarm signs, in many instances, it is reasonable to perform some inexpensive and noninvasive work-up to evaluate for an identifiable organic process (**Table 2**). These include blood tests such as a complete blood cell count, liver panel, inflammatory markers, and celiac screen. Tissue transglutaminase immunoglobulin A (IgA) is the most reliable and cost-effective marker for celiac disease.[23] It is important to check total IgA levels as well to avoid a false-negative TTG among those who are IgA deficient, who may be symptom-free. Rates of celiac are higher in those with selective IgA deficiency compared with the general

Table 2
Potential early or noninvasive testing

Serum	Stool	Urine	Imaging
CBC	Occult blood	Pregnancy	Abdominal ultrasound
LFT	Calprotectin	Urinalysis	Abdominal MRI
ESR	Infectious studies		
CRP	• Giardia		
TTG	• C difficile		
Total IgA	• Salmonella		
Lipase	• Shigella		
	• Campylobacter		

population.[24] Stool testing for occult blood is a low-cost and potentially high-yield test. Stool calprotectin is an increasingly important noninvasive biomarker in the evaluation of abdominal pain in children. Much like a sedimentation rate, it is a marker of inflammation. However, it is specific to the GI tract. Data suggest calprotectin can reliably distinguish IBS and functional abdominal pain from similarly presenting conditions such as inflammatory bowel disease.[25] For patients with prolonged diarrhea, it is important to test for treatable infectious processes such as Giardia or Clostridium difficile, which can cause chronic symptoms in the appropriate clinical setting.

International pediatric GI society guidelines recommend against routine testing for H pylori.[26] There is poor correlation between the presence H pylori and symptoms, in the absence of ulceration. Treatment does not necessarily result in symptom resolution. Serum testing for H pylori has poor sensitivity and specificity and cannot distinguish active from past infection.[27] When H pylori is suspected, as in the context of epigastric pain, nausea, and dyspepsia, upper endoscopy is the preferred method of testing. It confirms the diagnosis and evaluates for complications (ie, ulceration) related to H pylori, as well as for other conditions with similar presentations. Following treatment, noninvasive testing for H pylori via stool or breath are reliable, and are performed to ensure eradication.

Imaging such as abdominal ultrasound and abdominal MRI are at times indicated. However, for nonspecific or nonfocal abdominal pain, and when there is no specific clinical concern, they are lower yield. Radiation associated with abdominal computed tomography (CT) precludes their use in the pediatric population in all but the most concerning cases for acute surgical processes or when concern for kidney stone is high. Abdominal CT serves essentially no role in chronic abdominal pain in pediatrics.

Even when noninvasive studies are reassuring, endoscopy may be indicated. For example, approximately 20% of Crohn disease patients and 50% of ulcerative colitis patients with mild symptoms have normal laboratory findings at presentation.[28] In instances in which functioning or sleep is severely impaired, or when parental or child anxiety remains high, endoscopy plays a role. Normal findings reassure patients and families a more worrisome process is not missed.

Although ensuring a correct diagnosis is critical, one must balance against over-medicalizing. Achieving this balance is among the most difficult challenges faced by providers. Testing can be expensive and carries risk (eg bowel perforation or anesthesia side effects during endoscopy or radiation from imaging). Benign incidental findings may cause undue concern and lead to additional unnecessary studies. Testing may be counter-productive when it distracts from the true diagnosis, delaying appropriate therapy. Instead, when an FGID is highly suspected, it is important to counsel on this likelihood prior to work-up. Emphasizing a low pretest probability prepares families for normal results. When families are not prepared for this possibility at the onset, they may expect additional investigation, which leads to frustration when it is not indicated. Appropriate counseling is critical in the management of FGIDs.

TREATMENT

Treatment for functional abdominal pain and other FGIDs can be difficult. First and most important is establishing trust and a therapeutic rapport with patients and their families. Often these patients receive a message from caregivers or providers that the pain is in their head. They may be accused of attention seeking or school avoidance. However, it is important to recognize that functional abdominal pain is truly painful. Discounting these symptoms is counterproductive. Instead, it is important to sympathize and validate. It is equally helpful to counsel on the underlying nature of symptoms. Explaining the brain-gut axis in simple terms provides families with an understanding of the cause of symptoms. Patients and families who seek a more scientific understanding may benefit from selective discussion of some of the known and hypothesized pathophysiology detailed previously (eg, serotonin balance, immune system dysregulation potentially influenced by psychosocial stress). Providing this information in turn makes it easier for patients to accept treatment modalities focused on breaking out of the vicious cycle associated with functional abdominal pain (pain causes fear; fear worsens pain). Counseling alone may be sufficient in cases of mild FGIDs. Indeed, appropriate counseling and reassurance alone has been shown to be therapeutic.[29]

Even when symptoms are mild, medical practitioners should refer early to mental health providers, who play a critical role in treatment of FGIDs. Cognitive behavioral therapy (CBT) has demonstrated efficacy in the treatment of functional abdominal pain,[30,31] especially when this CBT is rooted in the psychoeducation detailed previously. Particularly effective CBT components in the treatment of FGIDs include thought restructuring to address negative attribution bias, guided relaxation strategies, as well as positive reinforcement paradigms focusing on rewarding functioning in the context of potentially ongoing pain. Family therapy plays an important role as well. Indeed, it is critical that parents validate symptoms as both real and in part emotionally based, establish and maintain positive reinforcement systems rewarding functioning, and detect and neutralize the possible role of secondary gain in symptom perpetuation. Psychiatrists, psychologists, and other pediatric mental health providers can also address conditions such as anxiety disorders and depressive disorders, which are often comorbid with FGIDs.[32] Abdominal pain may only be the somatic complaint tip of the iceberg.

Dietary changes play a role in the treatment of FGIDs. Even when celiac disease is excluded, some patients may be gluten-sensitive and respond to a gluten-free or gluten-restricted diet. Likewise, a diet low in FODMAP (fermentable, oligo-, di-, mono-saccharides and polyols) may be effective.[33] FODMAPs are poorly absorbed carbohydrates, which bypass digestion in the small intestine and are fermented by colonic bacteria. Byproducts of this process such as methane, carbon dioxide, and short chain fatty acids may induce symptoms. Lactose is a commonly encountered FODMAP, which may be particularly problematic among those with lactase deficiency. Practitioners should be mindful, however, in their prescription of restricted diets. Patients and families may overattribute FGID symptoms to dietary issues, which can distract from the treatment of underlying emotional distress. Nutritional deficiencies and disordered eating behaviors could potentially emerge secondary to prescribed or parentally pursued dietary restrictions.

Medicines, which tend to target specific symptoms, also play a role in the treatment of FGIDs. When patients describe painful spasms, it is reasonable to try antispasmodic agents such as dicyclomine or hyoscyamine, although data are lacking.[34] Peppermint oil is a natural antispasmodic, which has good evidence to support its use.[35,36] Probiotics may play a role in the treatment of FGIDs. Although probiotics can be expensive, they have benign side effect profiles, so at the least, will likely do no physiologic harm. For those with constipation, stool softeners such as polyethylene glycol, and stimulants such as senna or bisacodyl, are commonly employed. Newer agents lubiprostone[37] and linaclotide[38,39] may be used in constipation-type IBS, although these are not yet approved for children. Acid suppression medications, such as proton pump inhibiters and H2 blockers, are superior to placebo for epigastric abdominal pain, even in the absence of acid peptic disease or gastroesophageal reflux disease (GERD).[40] For these functional dyspepsia patients, or for those with episodic pain associated with abdominal migraine, cyproheptadine can be effective.[41,42] Side effects of this serotonin antagonist include increased appetite and fatigue, so it is particularly helpful in those who are underweight or those with insomnia. Unfortunately, it can interfere with antidepressant agents, which may also be used to treat FGIDs. Data among adult populations with FGIDs show benefit of antidepressant medications such as tricyclic antidepressants (TCAs) and selective serotonin reuptake inhibitors (SSRIs).[43] However, these findings have not been consistently replicated among children.[44] The potential utility in SSRIs for FGIDs is strengthened by the identification of comorbid anxiety disorders and/or depressive disorders. When such a comorbidity is identified, SSRIs are often preferred over TCAs because of reduced side effect profiles, increased safety in accidental or intentional ingestion, and increased efficacy with regard to the identified comorbid condition. Collaboration between medical and psychiatry providers is warranted to avoid polypharmacy and ensure an appropriate medication regimen.

SUMMARY

Functional abdominal pain and related FGIDs are commonly encountered by pediatricians, psychiatrists, psychologists, and other pediatric mental health providers. Somatic complaints are frequently a prominent presenting symptom of psychiatric disease such as anxiety and depression. In contrast, patients with inflammatory GI conditions such as celiac or inflammatory bowel disease may persist with symptoms, even when their inflammation is well controlled. Functional GI symptoms may be indistinguishable from identifiable organic GI disease, which poses a diagnostic challenge. Although it is critical to exclude a harmful process, it is likewise important to avoid unnecessary testing and maintain focus. FGIDs are not a diagnosis of exclusion, so minimal testing is required when suspicion is high. Nevertheless, testing may be appropriate to reassure families and providers that an otherwise identifiable organic process is not missed. The Rome criteria can help guide clinicians toward appropriate diagnosis and aid researchers in characterizing their study populations. More research is needed to help pharmacologic therapies in the treatment of FGIDs. Due to lackluster efficacy and a high placebo response rate, medications play a secondary role in the treatment of these conditions. Most important is appropriate counseling and reassurance rooted in education from medical and mental health providers. Optimal treatment of FGIDs requires collaboration among clinical services.

REFERENCES

1. Korterink JJ, Diederen K, Benninga MA, et al. Epidemiology of pediatric functional abdominal pain disorders: a meta-analysis. PLoS One 2015;10(5): e0126982.
2. Saps M, Seshadri R, Sztainberg M, et al. A prospective school-based study of abdominal pain and other common somatic complaints in children. J Pediatr 2009;154(3):322–6.
3. National ambulatory medical care survey: 2013 state and national summary tables. Available at: https://www.cdc.gov/nchs/data/ahcd/namcs_summary/2013_namcs_web_tables.pdf. Accessed August 16, 2017.
4. National Hospital Ambulatory Medical Care Survey: 2013 emergency department summary tables. Available at: https://www.cdc.gov/nchs/data/ahcd/nhamcs_emergency/2013__wedeb_tables.pdf. Accessed August 16, 2017.
5. Dhroove G, Chogle A, Saps M. A million-dollar work-up for abdominal pain: is it worth it? J Pediatr Gastroenterol Nutr 2010;51(5):579–83.
6. Drossman DA, Hasler WL. Rome IV-functional GI disorders: disorders of gut-brain interaction. Gastroenterology 2016;150(6):1257–61.
7. Barbara G, Cremon C, Carini G, et al. The immune system in irritable bowel syndrome. J Neurogastroenterol Motil 2011;17(4):349–59.
8. Hyams JS, Di Lorenzo C, Saps M, et al. Functional disorders: children and adolescents. Gastroenterology 2016. [Epub ahead of print].
9. Collins SM, Bercik P. The relationship between intestinal microbiota and the central nervous system in normal gastrointestinal function and disease. Gastroenterology 2009;136(6):2003–14.
10. Tillisch K, Labus J, Kilpatrick L, et al. Consumption of fermented milk product with probiotic modulates brain activity. Gastroenterology 2013;144(7):1394–401, 1401.e1-4.
11. Bennet SM, Ohman L, Simren M. Gut microbiota as potential orchestrators of irritable bowel syndrome. Gut Liver 2015;9(3):318–31.
12. McVey Neufeld KA, Perez-Burgos A, Mao YK, et al. The gut microbiome restores intrinsic and extrinsic nerve function in germ-free mice accompanied by changes in calbindin. Neurogastroenterol Motil 2015;27(5):627–36.
13. Wang B, Mao YK, Diorio C, et al. Luminal administration ex vivo of a live *Lactobacillus* species moderates mouse jejunal motility within minutes. FASEB J 2010; 24(10):4078–88.
14. Mayer EA, Savidge T, Shulman RJ. Brain-gut microbiome interactions and functional bowel disorders. Gastroenterology 2014;146(6):1500–12.
15. Zhang L, Song J, Hou X. Mast cells and irritable bowel syndrome: from the bench to the bedside. J Neurogastroenterol Motil 2016;22(2):181–92.
16. Barbara G, Wang B, Stanghellini V, et al. Mast cell-dependent excitation of visceral-nociceptive sensory neurons in irritable bowel syndrome. Gastroenterology 2007;132(1):26–37.
17. Mawdsley JE, Rampton DS. Psychological stress in IBD: new insights into pathogenic and therapeutic implications. Gut 2005;54(10):1481–91.
18. Gershon MD, Tack J. The serotonin signaling system: from basic understanding to drug development for functional GI disorders. Gastroenterology 2007;132(1): 397–414.

19. Gebhart GF. Visceral pain-peripheral sensitisation [review]. Gut 2000;47(Suppl 4): iv54–5 [discussion: iv58].

20. Halpin SJ, Ford AC. Prevalence of symptoms meeting criteria for irritable bowel syndrome in inflammatory bowel disease: systematic review and meta-analysis. Am J Gastroenterol 2012;107(10):1474–82.

21. Sainsbury A, Sanders DS, Ford AC. Prevalence of irritable bowel syndrome-type symptoms in patients with celiac disease: a meta-analysis. Clin Gastroenterol Hepatol 2013;11(4):359–65.e1.

22. Thabane M, Simunovic M, Akhtar-Danesh N, et al. An outbreak of acute bacterial gastroenteritis is associated with an increased incidence of irritable bowel syndrome in children. Am J Gastroenterol 2010;105(4):933–9.

23. Husby S, Koletzko S, Korponay-Szabó IR, et al. European Society for Pediatric Gastroenterology, Hepatology, and Nutrition guidelines for the diagnosis of coeliac disease. J Pediatr Gastroenterol Nutr 2012;54(1):136–60.

24. Chow MA, Lebwohl B, Reilly NR, et al. Immunoglobulin A deficiency in celiac disease. J Clin Gastroenterol 2012;46(10):850–4.

25. van Rheenen PF, Van de Vijver E, Fidler V. Faecal calprotectin for screening of patients with suspected inflammatory bowel disease: diagnostic meta-analysis. BMJ 2010;341:c3369.

26. Jones NL, Koletzko S, Goodman K, et al. Joint ESPGHAN/NASPGHAN guidelines for the management of *Helicobacter pylori* in children and adolescents (Update 2016). J Pediatr Gastroenterol Nutr 2017;64(6):991–1003.

27. Guarner J, Kalach N, Elitsur Y, et al. *Helicobacter pylori* diagnostic tests in children: review of the literature from 1999 to 2009. Eur J Pediatr 2010;169(1):15–25.

28. Mack DR, Langton C, Markowitz J, et al. Laboratory values for children with newly diagnosed inflammatory bowel disease. Pediatrics 2007;119(6):1113–9.

29. Kaptchuk TJ, Kelley JM, Conboy LA, et al. Components of placebo effect: randomised controlled trial in patients with irritable bowel syndrome. BMJ 2008; 336(7651):999–1003.

30. Huertas-Ceballos A, Logan S, Bennett C, et al. Pharmacological interventions for recurrent abdominal pain (RAP) and irritable bowel syndrome (IBS) in childhood. Cochrane Database Syst Rev 2008;(1):CD003017.

31. Zijdenbos IL, de Wit NJ, van der Heijden GJ, et al. Psychological treatments for the management of irritable bowel syndrome. Cochrane Database Syst Rev 2009;(1):CD006442.

32. Whitehead WE, Palsson O, Jones KR. Systematic review of the comorbidity of irritable bowel syndrome with other disorders: what are the causes and implications? Gastroenterology 2002;122(4):1140–56.

33. Staudacher HM, Whelan K. The low FODMAP diet: recent advances in understanding its mechanisms and efficacy in IBS. Gut 2017;66(8):1517–27.

34. Ruepert L, Quartero AO, de Wit NJ, et al. Bulking agents, antispasmodics and antidepressants for the treatment of irritable bowel syndrome. Cochrane Database Syst Rev 2011;(8):CD003460.

35. Cappello G, Spezzaferro M, Grossi L, et al. Peppermint oil (Mintoil) in the treatment of irritable bowel syndrome: a prospective double blind placebo-controlled randomized trial. Dig Liver Dis 2007;39(6):530–6.

36. Cash BD, Epstein MS, Shah SM. A novel delivery system of peppermint oil is an effective therapy for irritable bowel syndrome symptoms. Dig Dis Sci 2016;61(2): 560–71.

37. Drossman DA, Chey WD, Johanson JF, et al. Clinical trial: lubiprostone in patients with constipation-associated irritable bowel syndrome–results of two randomized, placebo-controlled studies. Aliment Pharmacol Ther 2009;29(3):329–41.
38. Chey WD, Lembo AJ, Lavins BJ, et al. Linaclotide for irritable bowel syndrome with constipation: a 26-week, randomized, double-blind, placebo-controlled trial to evaluate efficacy and safety. Am J Gastroenterol 2012;107(11):1702–12.
39. Rao S, Lembo AJ, Shiff SJ, et al. A 12-week, randomized, controlled trial with a 4-week randomized withdrawal period to evaluate the efficacy and safety of linaclotide in irritable bowel syndrome with constipation. Am J Gastroenterol 2012; 107(11):1714–24 [quiz: p.1725].
40. Pinto-Sanchez MI, Yuan Y, Bercik P, et al. Proton pump inhibitors for functional dyspepsia. Cochrane Database Syst Rev 2017;(3):CD011194.
41. Rodriguez L, Diaz J, Nurko S. Safety and efficacy of cyproheptadine for treating dyspeptic symptoms in children. J Pediatr 2013;163(1):261–7.
42. Worawattanakul M, Rhoads JM, Lichtman SN, et al. Abdominal migraine: prophylactic treatment and follow-up. J Pediatr Gastroenterol Nutr 1999;28(1):37–40.
43. Xie C, Tang Y, Wang Y, et al. Efficacy and safety of antidepressants for the treatment of irritable bowel syndrome: a meta-analysis. PLoS One 2015;10(8): e0127815.
44. Kaminski A, Kamper A, Thaler K, et al. Antidepressants for the treatment of abdominal pain-related functional gastrointestinal disorders in children and adolescents. Cochrane Database Syst Rev 2011;(7):CD008013.

Unraveling Diagnostic Uncertainty Surrounding Lyme Disease in Children with Neuropsychiatric Illness

Michael P. Koster, MD[a],*, Aris Garro, MD, MPH[b]

KEYWORDS

- Lyme disease • Neuroborreliosis • Neuropsychiatric • Neurocognitive
- Post-Lyme disease syndrome

KEY POINTS

- Lyme disease is a treatable condition that should be considered in the evaluation of patients with neuropsychiatric illness.
- Prolonged antibiotics, beyond the recommended standard treatment, are not indicated in Lyme disease.
- Only clinical syndromes consistent with Lyme disease should prompt testing.
- Symptoms of post-Lyme disease syndrome can be treated with symptom-directed care.

INTRODUCTION

Lyme disease is the most common vector-borne illness in the world, with most reports from North America and Europe. In 2015, there were 28,453 cases of confirmed Lyme disease, with 9616 probable cases in the United States. The annual incidence in endemic areas of the United States is 8.9 cases per 100,000 persons, with 5- to 10-year-old children comprising the largest affected group.[1] An understanding of the clinical manifestations of Lyme disease and diagnostic test performance is essential for the psychiatric provider to determine whether Lyme disease is playing a role in a given child's illness. In some patients, symptoms may continue after appropriate treatment, best described as post-Lyme disease syndrome. This is in contrast to the poorly defined term chronic Lyme disease, which perpetuates the misperception that infection persists after standard treatment. The symptoms of post-Lyme disease syndrome

[a] Department of Pediatrics, Alpert Medical School of Brown University, Rhode Island Hospital – Hasbro Children's Hospital, 593 Eddy Street, Providence, RI 02903, USA; [b] Division of Pediatric Emergency Medicine, Alpert Medical School of Brown University, Rhode Island Hospital - Hasbro Children's Hospital, 125 Whipple Street, UEMF Suite-3rd Floor, Providence, RI 02908, USA
* Corresponding author.
E-mail address: mkoster@lifespan.org

Child Adolesc Psychiatric Clin N Am 27 (2018) 27–36
http://dx.doi.org/10.1016/j.chc.2017.08.010
1056-4993/18/© 2017 Elsevier Inc. All rights reserved.

childpsych.theclinics.com

are typically nonspecific and involve multiple organ systems including, joints, muscles, nerves, brain, and heart.

ROLE OF THE PSYCHIATRIC PROVIDER

Meaningful and empathetic engagement is paramount to establishing a trusting therapeutic alliance and empowering parents to make informed decisions. Collaboration with the primary care practitioner in developing a thoughtful approach to a complicated diagnosis can reduce unintended or inappropriate testing, as well as misinterpretation of test results. In post-Lyme disease syndrome, the clinical psychiatrist is in a good position to offer therapy for neuropathic pain (eg, gabapentin), sleep disturbances (eg, tricyclic antidepressants), or coexistent mood disorders (eg, selective serotonin uptake inhibitors). Clinical psychiatrists are also well equipped to address physical complaints such as malaise, headache, or anxiety with conventional interventions that provide coping skills including cognitive behavioral therapy, mind/body techniques, and recommendations for structured physical activity.

PRESENTATIONS OF LYME DISEASE

Lyme disease is a tick-borne infection caused by *Borrelia burgdorferi.*[2] The stages of Lyme disease are early localized, early disseminated, and late. Unlike other infectious diseases, the manifestations of Lyme disease do not necessarily present in a progressive linear fashion. Most children (>90%) present with early localized disease, which is identifiable by a single, circular, expanding lesion measuring at least 5 cm and known as erythema migrans (EM).[3] This macular lesion expands over days, often with central-clearing, and occasionally resembles a targetoid lesion (**Fig. 1**). Clinicians in areas where Lyme disease is endemic become adept at identifying EM lesions.

Lyme disease often presents with multiple EM lesions, appearing days to weeks after a single EM lesion. Lyme neuroborreliosis (LNB; 3%–5% of infected patients) is another manifestation of early disseminated Lyme disease and presents with either a facial nerve palsy, meningitis, or both.[2–4] Lyme disease-associated facial nerve palsy presents as a unilateral facial droop that affects the forehead, eyebrow, nasolabial fold, and lips. Occasionally the facial droop will be bilateral, which is highly suggestive for Lyme disease in endemic areas. Lyme meningitis can present with the classic

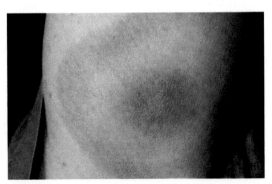

Fig. 1. Erythema migrans lesion. (*From* Centers for Disease Control and Prevention (CDC). Lyme disease: signs and symptoms. Lyme disease rashes and look-alikes. Available at: https://www.cdc.gov/lyme/signs_symptoms/rashes.html. Accessed July 17, 2017.)

findings of headache and neck stiffness, but these manifestations are often insidious and less pronounced than meningitis caused by bacteria or viruses. Increased intracranial pressure and papilledema, sometimes associated with an abducens palsy (causing diplopia and less commonly esotropia), is well described in children with Lyme meningitis. Optic neuritis can present with visual disturbances including vision loss.

Lyme carditis is another manifestation of early disseminated Lyme disease, occurring in less than 1% of children.[2–4] Lyme carditis can present as first-, second-, or rarely third-degree heart block on electrocardiogram (ECG). This heart block is generally self-limited and rarely requires advanced intervention such as cardiac pacing.

Arthritis, the chief presentation of late disease (5%–10% of infected patients), typically occurs months after infection.[2–4] Monoarticular infection of the knee is most common, where there is impressive swelling with only mild-to-moderate pain and minimal erythema overlying the joint. Ten percent of patients with arthritis develop chronic noninfectious arthritis. Polyneuropathy with radiculoneuritis (Bannwarth Syndrome) is especially rare in children but should be suspected in endemic European areas when symptoms include muscle weakness, neuralgia, and/or paresthesias. Late neurologic diseases including encephalomyelitis or encephalopathy are extremely rare in pediatrics given better detection and earlier treatment, but if they occur, could mimic psychosis.[4]

Case reports of neuropsychological manifestations of Lyme disease that are of special interest to psychiatrists include: Alice in Wonderland syndrome (sensation that things are getting larger and smaller), Tourette syndrome, acute delirium, catatonia, psychosis, and stroke mimics such as aphasia.[5–9] Although these case reports demonstrate that Lyme disease can present with atypical neuropsychiatric manifestations, it is important to note they are rare and can typically be distinguished by other signs and symptoms of Lyme disease, such as an accompanying facial palsy. Additionally, objective findings can help to make the diagnosis of Lyme disease, including positive Lyme serology with lymphocytic pleocytosis in the cerebrospinal fluid, or intrathecal production of Lyme antibody. MRI may show nonspecific white matter changes with increased signal on T2 and FLAIR postcontrast sequences.[2]

NEUROPSYCHIATRIC AND CLINICAL OUTCOMES IN CHILDREN WITH LYME DISEASE

Given the neurotropism of *Borrelia burgdorferi,* it is not surprising that patients could experience neuropsychiatric symptoms after infection including sleep disturbance, memory problems, and mood changes. What is difficult to determine is whether these symptoms are a direct result of Lyme disease infection, or whether they occur with similar frequency in the general population, in which case they coexist with Lyme disease but are not direct sequelae. In practice, it does not matter, as further antibiotic treatment does not improve outcomes, leaving symptom-directed care as the mainstay in both scenarios. In other words, after the child receives appropriate treatment for Lyme disease, the focus should be on improving the child's emotional and psychological well-being and quality of life using standard therapeutic techniques familiar to psychiatrists.

Several studies have examined neuropsychiatric symptoms in children treated for Lyme disease compared with the general population. In 1999, Adams and colleagues[10] performed a 4-year follow-up of patients with Lyme disease compared with case-matched siblings without Lyme disease. They found similar intelligence, processing speed, fine-motor dexterity, executive functioning, memory, and depression in children who had been treated for Lyme disease compared with matched healthy siblings. Children with treated Lyme disease only had poorer performance on a single short-term visual memory test, but this was felt to be of little clinical significance. Parents of children in the Lyme disease group expressed subjective beliefs that their children did not have a progressively deteriorating course affecting academic performance or psychosocial domains.

Vazquez, and colleagues[11] identified the risk of neurocognitive deficits in children who had Lyme disease-associated facial palsy compared with healthy controls. They found similar long-term neuropsychological and health outcomes between children with Lyme disease-associated facial palsy and healthy controls, except for statistically significant differences in the frequency of neck pain (16 vs 1%), behavioral changes (16 vs 2%), pain in joints or muscles (21 vs 5%), numbness or funny sensations in nerves (12 vs 2%), and memory problems (9 vs 1%). They did not find differences between groups with respect to fatigue, swollen joints, headaches, school attendance and performance, exercise tolerance, appetite, sleeping, performance of household chores, naming objects, word recall, judgment, academic performance, organization of ideas, or gym attendance. Interestingly when parents and patients were asked whether they thought their Lyme disease had been cured, 79% believed their Lyme was cured; 9% believed it was not cured (citing as reasons: headaches, fatigue, joint redness or popping, suspicion that disease can lay dormant in the body), and 12% were unsure if it was cured. Overall subjects had excellent perceived treatment outcomes.

A more recent study looking at long-term clinical outcomes in children after LNB was performed by Skogman and colleagues[12] in 2012. In this study, 84 Swedish children with Lyme disease and 84 matched controls were evaluated by physical examination and a structured questionnaire. They found no difference between Lyme disease patients and healthy controls with respect to nonspecific symptoms such as headache, neck pain, sleep disturbances, fatigue, poor appetite, memory, concentration problems, and school performance. They did find differences in residual facial palsy (8 vs 0%), vertigo (7 vs 1%), and pain, numbness, or weakness of limbs (7 vs 1%).

Finally, Nadelman and colleagues[13] performed screening of adult patients admitted to an inpatient psychiatric unit in an endemic area. Of the 517 patients screened, only 1 patient was positive by EIA and was negative by immunoblotting. This study demonstrated that Lyme disease is a rare comorbid condition in patients with common psychiatric conditions.

DIAGNOSTIC TESTING FOR LYME DISEASE

The pretest probability of Lyme disease must be known to appropriately interpret the results of Lyme disease tests. This is difficult when children have symptoms that occur in Lyme disease, but have low specificity for Lyme disease. For example, headache, fever, myalgias, and fatigue are frequent symptoms of Lyme disease, but are also found in a multitude of other illnesses. In children with these isolated, nonspecific symptoms, the pretest probability of Lyme disease will be low. The tests for Lyme disease, even when positive, are not accurate enough to change the post-test probability of Lyme disease, and thus will frequently result in false positives (**Fig. 2**). Diagnostic tests for Lyme disease should only be performed when children present with known clinical symptoms that increase the pretest probability of Lyme disease during seasons in which Lyme disease is endemic.

There are 2 scenarios that are highly specific for Lyme disease. The first is an EM lesion. A clinical diagnosis of EM by a clinician who is experienced in recognizing these

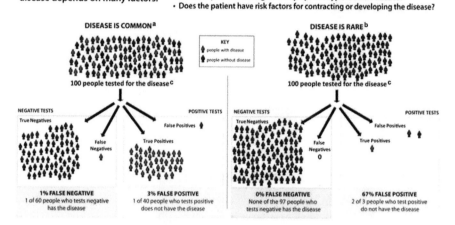

Fig. 2. Test results for infectious diseases. [a] Forty percent of patients in this area have the disease. [b] One percent of patients in this area have this disease. [c] Test specificity = 98% (high) and test sensitivity = 98% (high). (*From* Centers for Disease Control and Prevention (CDC). Lyme disease: resources for clinicians. Available at: https://www.cdc.gov/lyme/resources/testresults_remediated.pdf. Accessed July 17, 2017.)

lesions is sufficient for diagnosing early localized Lyme disease, and serologic testing should not be performed, as it is unreliable at this stage with frequent false negatives. Bilateral peripheral facial nerve palsy (simultaneous or sequential) is also specific for Lyme disease in endemic regions. Other clinical symptomatologies associated with higher pretest probabilities of Lyme disease include: unilateral peripheral facial nerve palsy, meningitis, carditis (heart block), and arthritis. Patients with facial palsy, lymphocytic pleocytosis in cerebrospinal fluid, heart block of any degree on ECG, or arthritis who live or travel to endemic areas should undergo serologic Lyme testing.

The seasonality of Lyme disease is important, because in the climes in which *B Burgdorferi* is endemic, the vectors of transmission (*Ixodes subspecies* ticks) are generally encountered between April and December.[1] Testing for most Lyme disease manifestations should be limited to these months, with the exception of arthritis, which is a late manifestation of Lyme disease and can present outside of the endemic months.

Serologic testing is the current gold standard for the diagnosis of Lyme disease. In North America, a 2-tier serologic testing system with good sensitivity (70%–100%) and specificity (>95%) is used.[14] Enzyme immunoassays (EIAs) detect Lyme-specific antibodies quantitatively (highly sensitive), and if positive or equivocal, a confirmatory Western immunoblot assay should be performed (highly specific). Because antibodies from previous *B Burgdorferi* infection can persist indefinitely even after adequate treatment, a test that is positive by immunoglobulin M (IgM) alone (negative IgG) is a false positive if symptoms have been present for longer than 30 days, because IgG antibody formation would be expected by that time also (**Fig. 3**).[15]

Two-tier Testing for Lyme Disease

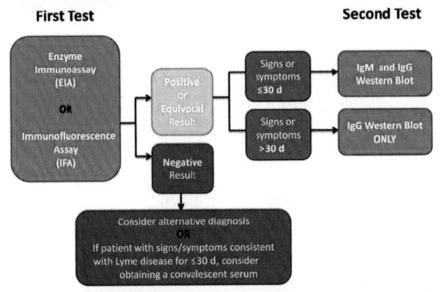

Fig. 3. The 2-tier TESTING DECISION TREE describes the steps required to properly test for Lyme disease. The first required test is the EIA or immunofluorescence assay (IFA). If this test yields negative results, the provider should consider an alternative diagnosis, or in cases where the patient with has had symptoms for no more than 30 days, the provider may treat the patient and follow with a convalescent serum. If the first test yields positive or equivocal results, 2 options are available. If the patient has had symptoms for less than or equal to 30 days, an IgM Western Blot is performed; if the patient has had symptoms for more than 30 days, the IgG Western Blot is performed. The IgM should not be used if the patient has been ill for more than 30 days. (*From* Centers for Disease Control and Prevention (CDC). Lyme disease: resources for clinicians. Available at: https://www.cdc.gov/lyme/resources/twotieredtesting.pdf. Accessed July 17, 2017.)

Other diagnostic tests for Lyme disease have been described, but at present are not included in guidelines for the diagnosis of Lyme disease in the United States. In Europe, an antibody index of Lyme-specific immunoglobulins in the spinal fluid relative to the serum is used, but it has not been widely adopted in the United States, because local antibody production is less consistent in US patients with neuroborreliosis.[16] Polymerase chain reaction tests to detect *B Burgdorferi* have proven useful from synovial fluid (80% sensitive), but not in cerebrospinal fluid (50% sensitive). Promising new tests involving C6, host RNA response, and metabolomics are being developed but are not currently widely used in the United States.[17]

Nonvalidated Testing

Other testing modalities have been developed but not yet validated for the diagnosis of Lyme disease. The US Centers for Disease Control and Prevention have issued statements against the use of these tests. Specific examples include but are not limited to

Capture assays for antigens in urine
B Burgdorferi culture
Immunofluorescence staining

Cell sorting of cell wall-deficient or cystic forms of *B burgdorferi*
Lymphocyte transformation tests
Quantitative CD57 lymphocyte assays
Reverse Western blots
In-house criteria for interpretation of immunoblots
Measurements of antibodies in synovial fluid
Western blot tests without a positive EIA[18]

Unfortunately, these tests are available commercially and are often used to test children, resulting in misdiagnosis. Steere and colleagues[19] found that of 788 patients referred to their clinic for Lyme disease, 452 patients (57%) had an illness other than Lyme disease. Of these patients, 203 (45%) had multiple positive studies from outside laboratories but were negative in the standardized laboratory.

TREATMENT OF LYME DISEASE

The Infectious Diseases Society of America has published guidelines for the diagnosis and treatment of Lyme disease, with defined durations of antibiotic treatment for the various presentations of Lyme disease. Additionally, randomized controlled trials demonstrate that prolonged antibiotics for the treatment of post-Lyme disease syndrome are not effective in reducing chronic musculoskeletal pain or neurocognitive symptoms associated with post-Lyme disease syndrome.[20–24] Neither microbiological nor molecular evidence for persistent *B borgdoferi* was found in any of the patients enrolled in these trials. Most importantly, the risks of unnecessary antibiotics are highlighted in case reports, including fatalities from acquired *Clostridium difficile* and *Candidida parapsilosis* infections in patients receiving prolonged antibiotic treatment for presumed Lyme disease.[25,26]

Unconventional Treatment

Unfortunately, many patients with subjective nonspecific symptoms who believe they are suffering from a chronic infection with Lyme disease are treated with unproven, nonantimicrobial treatments for Lyme disease. The scope of this problem was reported by Lantos and colleagues,[27] who identified over 30 alternative treatments offered on the Internet. Many unproven therapies had the potential to cause harm. For example, 1 treatment included deliberate inoculation of malaria into Lyme disease patients. The rise of such alternative treatments is often directed toward patients suffering from symptoms of post-Lyme disease syndrome. This is important to the psychiatrist, because patients will seek care for symptoms such as depression, fatigue, anxiety, and distress form residual physical dysfunction (eg, arthritis, residual facial palsy). Psychiatrists have a key role in treating these patients and potentially preventing the use of alternative treatments that will be at best useless, and at worst harmful.

ASSIMILATING DATA AND APPROACH TO CLINICAL SCENARIOS

The following are 3 clinical scenarios a clinical psychiatrist may encounter involving the differential diagnosis of Lyme disease.

Clinical Scenario One

Presentation

A teenager under your care for a mood disorder reports difficulty in school, trouble with memory, fatigue, poor sleep, and exercise intolerance. The mother of the child has been researching symptoms on the Internet and believes that her child could be suffering from Lyme disease. She would like to have her child tested and potentially treated for Lyme disease.

Resolution

In this scenario, a teenager who has not been previously diagnosed or treated for Lyme disease presents with parental concern. The patient does not present with a clinical scenario that is consistent with Lyme disease (low specificity). The likelihood of a false-positive test is higher than a true positive when the pretest probability falls below 20%, and the risks of unnecessary antibiotics are significant. It is possible that discussion with the family can help the patient and parents better understand the lack of association with nonspecific symptoms, and the need for objective clinical findings to prompt testing. In this case, Lyme disease testing should not be performed.

Clinical Scenario Two

Presentation

For the past 6 months you have been treating a young adolescent for depression in your clinic. The patient was previously healthy until having Lyme meningitis with facial palsy 2 years ago. The patient was appropriately treated with parenteral ceftriaxone for 14 days. There is some residual facial nerve palsy, and the patient continues complaining of fatigue and poor concentration. During a hospitalization for a major depressive episode, it comes to the clinicians' attention that the patient has been on daily oral doxycycline for the past 6 months. The admitting team is questioning the need for ongoing antibiotics during the acute inpatient admission.

Resolution

In this scenario, a patient is experiencing residual facial nerve palsy, a well-described sequela of LNB. This is stressful for the patient, as it is likely to impact social interactions and self-esteem. Psychiatric treatment should be focused on the patient's mental health as it relates to this sequela. Further treatment with antibiotics will not improve the facial palsy. It is understandable that parents want to have hope for the treatment of their child, but the lack of evidence for prolonged antibiotic treatment suggests that chronic infection is not the cause. A discussion about the risks and benefits of treatment are critical for empowering the family to make an educated decision. In this case, antibiotics should not be continued.

Clinical Scenario Three

Presentation

A school-aged child in your treatment for behavioral outburst in school also complains of intermittent fevers, headaches, neck and joint pains, fatigue, and poor academic performance. The child had special testing for Lyme disease finding an elevated CD57 lymphocyte and positive expanded immunoblot assay. The parents are confused about the testing and wanted to discuss with you prior to initiating the prescribed treatment of azithromycin, hydroxychloroquine, and mefloquine.

Resolution

In this scenario, the patient does have a clinical presentation that is consistent with Lyme disease (meningitis), but has come to you with invalid testing. The key to this case is to perform 2-tier Lyme serology and a lumbar puncture to definitively establish the diagnosis. In addition, the child is being offered nonstandard treatment, which could result in inadequate treatment (if he does indeed have Lyme disease) and a higher rate of adverse events. In this case, testing in a regulated laboratory should be offered, and if positive, a standardized treatment should be prescribed.

RECOMMENDATIONS FOR CLINICAL PSYCHIATRISTS

Test patients who present with a clinical syndrome consistent with Lyme disease. Always used 2-tier serologic testing from regulated laboratories and appreciate the importance of test interpretation, including false positive immunoblots by IgM alone, when symptoms are present longer than 1 month. Recognize appropriate antibiotic treatment; after a child has received sufficient treatment, further use of antibiotics to treat Lyme disease are not indicated. Manage patients who have post-Lyme disease syndrome with standard symptom-directed pharmacologic and nonpharmacological interventions in a multidisciplinary, empathetic, and evidence-based manner.

SUMMARY

Psychiatric providers play an important role in identifying children with neuropsychiatric symptoms that could be caused by Lyme disease, as well as in the care of patients with post-Lyme disease syndrome. Patients suffering from psychiatric symptoms, whether attributable to Lyme disease or coexisting with Lyme disease, require compassionate providers who are familiar with an evidence-based approach to Lyme disease. This familiarity empowers clinicians to know whom to test, what tests to send, how to interpret test results, which treatment to provide (or not provide), and how to approach persistent symptoms after Lyme disease has been appropriately treated.

REFERENCES

1. Centers for Disease Control and Prevention - Lyme disease statistics. Available at: https://www.cdc.gov/lyme/stats/index.html. Accessed July 17, 2017.
2. Stanek G, Wormser GP, Gray J, et al. Lyme borreliosis. Lancet 2012;379(9814): 461–73.
3. Gerber MA, Shapiro ED, Burke GS, et al. Lyme disease in children in southeastern Connecticut. Pediatric Lyme Disease Study Group. N Engl J Med 1996;335(17):1270–4.
4. Wormser G-P, Dattwyler R-J, Shapiro E-D, et al. The clinical assessment, treatment, and prevention of lyme disease, human granulocytic anaplasmosis, and babesiosis: clinical practice guidelines by the Infectious Diseases Society of America. Clin Infect Dis 2006;43(9):1089–134.
5. Binalsheikh IM, Griesemer D, Wang S, et al. Lyme neuroborreliosis presenting as Alice in Wonderland syndrome. Pediatr Neurol 2012;46(3):185–6.
6. Schwenkenbecher P, Pul R, Wurster U, et al. Common and uncommon neurological manifestations of neuroborreliosis leading to hospitalization. BMC Infect Dis 2017;17(1):90.
7. Baumann M, Birnbacher R, Koch J, et al. Uncommon manifestations of neuroborreliosis in children. Eur J Paediatr Neurol 2010;14(3):274–7.
8. Sokolov AA, Lienhard R, Du Pasquier R, et al. Acute Lyme neuroborreliosis with transient hemiparesis and aphasia. Ann Emerg Med 2015;66(1):60–4.
9. Riedel M, Straube A, Schwarz MJ, et al. Lyme disease presenting as Tourette's syndrome. Lancet 1998;351(9100):418–9.
10. Adams WV, Rose CD, Eppes SC, et al. Long-term cognitive effects of Lyme disease in children. Appl Neuropsychol 1999;6(1):39–45.

11. Vazquez M, Sparrow SS, Shapiro ED. Long-term neuropsychologic and health outcomes of children with facial nerve palsy attributable to Lyme disease. Pediatrics 2003;112(2):e93–7.

12. Skogman BH, Glimåker K, Nordwall M, et al. Long-term clinical outcome after Lyme neuroborreliosis in childhood. Pediatrics 2012;130(2):262–9.

13. Nadelman RB, Herman E, Wormser GP. Screening for Lyme disease in hospitalized psychiatric patients: prospective serosurvey in an endemic area. Mt Sinai J Med 1997;64(6):409–12.

14. Moore A, Nelson C, Molins C, et al. Current guidelines, common clinical pitfalls, and future directions for laboratory diagnosis of Lyme disease, United States. Emerg Infect Dis 2017;22(7):1169–77.

15. Lantos PM, Lipsett SC, Nigrovic LE. False positive Lyme disease IgM immunoblots in children. J Pediatr 2016;174:267–9.e1.

16. Steere AC, Berardi VP, Weeks KE, et al. Evaluation of the intrathecal antibody response to Borrelia burgdorferi as a diagnostic test for lyme neuroborreliosis. J Infect Dis 1990;161(6):1203–9.

17. Lipsett SC, Pollock NR, Branda JA, et al. The positive predictive value of Lyme ELISA for the diagnosis of Lyme disease in children. Pediatr Infect Dis J 2015; 34(11):1260–2.

18. Nelson CA. Concerns regarding a new culture method for Borrelia burgdorferi not approved for the diagnosis of Lyme disease. MMWR Morb Mortal Wkly Rep 2014; 63(15):333.

19. Steere AC. The overdiagnosis of Lyme disease. JAMA 1993;269(14):1812–6.

20. Klempner MS, Hu LT, Evans J, et al. Two controlled trials of antibiotic treatment in patients with persistent symptoms and a history of Lyme disease. N Engl J Med 2001;345(2):85–92.

21. Kaplan RF, Trevino RP, Johnson GM, et al. Cognitive function in post-treatment Lyme disease do additional antibiotics help? Neurology 2003;60(12):1916–22.

22. Krupp LB, Hyman LG, Grimson R, et al. Study and treatment of post Lyme disease (STOP-LD): a randomized double masked clinical trial. Neurology 2003; 60(12):1923–30.

23. Fallon BA, Keilp JG, Corbera KM, et al. A randomized, placebo-controlled trial of repeated IV antibiotic therapy for Lyme encephalopathy. Neurology 2008;70(13 PART 1):992–1003.

24. Berende A, ter Hofstede HJM, Vos FJ, et al. Randomized trial of longer-term therapy for symptoms attributed to Lyme disease. N Engl J Med 2016;374(13): 1209–20.

25. Patel R, Grogg KL, Edwards WD, et al. Death from inappropriate therapy for Lyme disease. Clin Infect Dis 2000;31(4):1107–9.

26. Holzbauer SM, Kemperman MM, Lynfield R. Death due to community-associated clostriudium difficile in a women receiving prolonged antibiotic therapy for suspected Lyme disease. Clin Infect Dis 2010;51(3):369–70.

27. Lantos PM, Shapiro ED, Auwaerter PG, et al. Unorthodox alternative therapies marketed to treat lyme disease. Clin Infect Dis 2015;60(12):1776–82.

Evaluation and Management of Autoimmune Encephalitis
A Clinical Overview for the Practicing Child Psychiatrist

GenaLynne C. Mooneyham, MD, MS[a,b,]*, William Gallentine, DO[c], Heather Van Mater, MD, MS[d]

KEYWORDS

- Autoimmune encephalitis • Autoimmune brain disorders • Antineuronal antibodies
- Anti-NMDA • Limbic encephalitis

KEY POINTS

- Autoimmune encephalitis often presents with neuropsychiatric symptoms, including but not limited to cognitive decline, paranoia, hypervigilance, sensory perceptual disturbances, and personality changes.
- Child psychiatrists must become familiar with autoimmune encephalitis because they may be the initial evaluator of children presenting with what may be otherwise misconstrued as purely psychiatric symptoms.
- The treatment of autoimmune encephalitis often includes immunomodulatory therapies to achieve symptom resolution or improvement.
- Child psychiatrists may be called on to advocate for their patients within the larger system to obtain the multidisciplinary evaluations necessary for treating autoimmune encephalitis.
- Residual symptoms of autoimmune encephalitis often require treatment aimed at symptom reduction with ongoing management even in the postinflammatory period.

The authors have no conflicts of interest to disclose.
[a] Department of Psychiatry, Division of Child and Family Mental Health and Developmental Neurosciences, Duke University, Durham, NC, USA; [b] Autoimmune Brain Disease Program, Department of Pediatrics, Duke University, Durham, NC, USA; [c] Autoimmune Brain Disease Program, Department of Pediatrics, Neurology Division, Duke University, Durham, NC, USA; [d] Autoimmune Brain Disease Program, Department of Pediatrics, Rheumatology Division, Duke University, Durham, NC, USA
* Corresponding author. Department of Child Psychiatry, Duke University Children's Hospital and Health Center, 2301 Erwin Road, Durham, NC 27710.
E-mail address: Genalynne.mooneyham@duke.edu

Child Adolesc Psychiatric Clin N Am 27 (2018) 37–52
http://dx.doi.org/10.1016/j.chc.2017.08.011
1056-4993/18/© 2017 Elsevier Inc. All rights reserved.

Abbreviations	
Anti-NMDAR	Anti–N-methyl-$_D$-aspartate receptor
CSF	Cerebrospinal fluid
EEG	Electroencephalograph
GAD 65	Glutamic acid decarboxylase 65
HE	Hashimoto's encephalopathy
IV	Intravenous
IVIG	Intravenous immunoglobulin
LE	Limbic encephalitis

INTRODUCTION

The field of neuroimmunology has expanded drastically over the past decade with the recognition and categorization of antineuronal antibodies within the central nervous system. Although the diagnosis of autoimmune encephalitis dates back to the 1970s, it was only in 2005 when the first specific antibody subtype, anti–N-methyl-$_D$-aspartate receptor (anti-NMDAR), was identified by Dr Josep Dalmua and his team.[1] Since that time, the number of known antibodies has substantially increased.[2] Many investigators in neuroimmunology hypothesize that there are far more antibodies yet to be identified. These antineuronal antibodies have been linked with neuropsychiatric symptoms including but not limited to the abrupt onset of personality changes, sensory perceptual disturbances, functional declines, and cognitive dulling.[3,4]

Autoimmune encephalitis is a broad diagnostic category that describes the subacute onset of neuropsychiatric symptoms whose etiology is linked with the clinical sequelae of the inflammatory response. The production of antibodies within the central nervous system or the periphery may be the result of molecular mimicry after an infectious process, systemic autoimmune disease(s), neoplasms, and/or paraneoplastic processes. Although the categorization of these antibodies is an ongoing effort, so too is the work of providing a meaningful nomenclature across the fields of psychiatry, neurology, rheumatology, and immunology.

DEFINITION OF AUTOIMMUNE ENCEPHALITIS

Encephalitis is any inflammation of the brain. There are many causes of encephalitis, of which autoimmune encephalitis is one. Autoimmune encephalitis may be best conceptualized as an umbrella term that includes several disease types. These subgroups are based on whether the presenting autoantibody is targeting the cell surface proteins, intracellular synaptic proteins, intracellular antigens, or is linked to a known paraneoplastic process.[5] In general, adults with autoimmune encephalitis diagnoses have a higher rate of association with paraneoplastic processes as compared with the child and adolescent population. According to Dalmau and colleagues, the diagnosis of autoimmune encephalitis no longer relies on the response to immunotherapy nor does it rely on a particular antibody status.[6] The topic of seronegative autoimmune encephalitis is discussed elsewhere in this article. Symptoms routinely seen in the active phase of autoimmune encephalitis include agitation, psychosis, catatonic features, delirium, seizures, changes in speech or mutism, and hallucinations. During the progression of disease, patients may begin to exhibit abnormal involuntary motor movements, respiratory compromise, decreased responsiveness progressing to coma, and autonomic dysregulation.

Diagnosis

The variability of symptoms both across and within subtypes of autoimmune encephalitis make diagnosing these conditions difficult. A high index of suspicion is required when evaluating children with new onset of neurologic and psychiatric symptoms to ensure prompt diagnosis and treatment. Recent efforts have focused on recognizing possible autoimmune encephalitis as a clinical diagnosis independent from antibody status. This measure is critical to ensure that patients start on first-line treatment even while awaiting antineuronal antibody testing given that earlier treatment is associated with improved outcomes.[3,4,6] In addition, experts recognize it is unlikely that all of the pathologic antineuronal antibodies have been discovered,[7,8] and that limiting treatment only to those who have a known antibody will exclude many patients with autoimmune encephalitis who would equally benefit from immunotherapy.[2,3,6]

Suspected Autoimmune Encephalitis

When children present with an acute to subacute onset of new neurologic and/or psychiatric symptoms spanning multiple domains, providers should consider autoimmune encephalitis in the differential (**Table 1**). The hallmark of autoimmune encephalitis is the progression of symptoms over days to months. Symptoms may include cognitive decline, memory impairment, movement disorders, seizures, sleep disturbances, language regression, behavior changes, developmental regression, psychosis, anxiety, and obsessive–compulsive disorder symptoms.[9,10] Initial evaluations will vary depending on the patient's primary symptoms. Children with new onset seizures who seem otherwise well may have a more limited evaluation, whereas those presenting with rapidly progressive encephalopathy will have a more extensive evaluation at the start. The complexity of these conditions and the changing symptomatology over time requires providers to remain vigilant.

Probable Autoimmune Encephalitis

The term "probable autoimmune encephalitis" is used to describe children with a clinical presentation consistent with autoimmune encephalitis, including acute to subacute onset of neuropsychiatric symptoms involving multiple domains, whose initial evaluation supports a noninfectious inflammatory process. The diagnosis requires that other etiologies have been excluded, including infectious, metabolic, genetic, and other syndromes. Paraclinical features of autoimmune encephalitis include MRI changes, elevated inflammatory parameters, cerebrospinal fluid (CSF) pleocytosis, CSF oligoclonal bands, changes on the electroencephalograph (EEG), and other serologies consistent with autoimmunity.[5,6,11,12] Imaging changes on MRI range from

Table 1	
Clinical features suggestive of autoimmune encephalitis	
Suggestive Features	**Features That Are Not Suggestive**
Abrupt onset	Chronic symptoms or indolent course
Rapid decline	Plateau in symptoms
Autonomic instability	
Enuresis/encopresis	No impairment in activities of daily living
Delirium ← → Catatonia	
Cognitive dulling	Maintaining cognitive capabilities
Gait/balance disturbances	Lack of fine/gross motor impairments
Multifocal drug resistant epilepsy	
Symptoms present in all environments	Environmental specific symptoms only
Multiple domains involved in symptoms	Solely psychiatric symptoms

normal findings to hyperintensities on T2-weighted or fluid-attenuated inversion recovery sequences to (less commonly) enhancing lesions or abnormalities on diffusion weighted imaging. Computed tomography scans are not sensitive for the inflammatory changes in autoimmune encephalitis.[2] EEGs are helpful to document seizures or slowing (focal or diffuse) that can support the diagnosis of an encephalopathy.

Initial Workup of Autoimmune Encephalitis

Consensus regarding a single diagnostic battery for autoimmune encephalitis has not yet been established. However, the list of laboratories, imaging, and ancillary studies in **Table 2** may be considered. Given the probability that immunomodulatory agents will be required if an autoimmune encephalitis is diagnosed, it is imperative to rule out infectious causes first. It can be difficult to differentiate between an acute encephalitis, a postinfectious encephalitis, and the possibility of an autoimmune encephalitis. Unfortunately, the disease trajectory itself often becomes an important diagnostic data point. A postinfectious encephalitis can resolve quickly and may not require escalation of immunomodulatory therapies, whereas an autoimmune encephalitis process will often show symptom progression without treatment.

Known Antibodies Associated with Autoimmune Encephalitis

Early treatment is essential and has been found to be one of the most significant predictors of a favorable outcome. The outcomes and treatment of autoimmune encephalitis may vary somewhat by subtype.

Table 2
Potential workup

Serum Tests	CSF Tests	Imaging	Ancillary Studies
CBC with differential	Opening pressure	MRI brain	Strep swab
CMP	Cell count	EEG routine	Throat culture
ANA	Glucose	Video EEG	Respiratory viral panel
Antithyroid antibody	Protein	PET scan	Mycoplasma swab
panel	Gram stain	MRA	24-h urine copper
Thyroid profile	Culture		Neuropsychological
Serum AE antibody panel[a]	ACE level		testing
Anticardiolipin antibody	CSF AE antibody panel[a]		Testicular/ovarian US
Anti-beta 2 glycoprotein	Oligoclonal bands/IgG		
Lupus anticoagulant	index		
ESR, CRP	Infectious workup (VZV,		
VonWillebrand factor	HSV, HHV-6)		
antigen			
Anti Sm, Ro, La antibody			
ACE level			
Anti-DNAse B			
ASO titer			
Mycoplasma IgG/IgM			
C3, C4			
Serum immunoglobulins			
Serum copper			
Creatine kinase			

Abbreviations: ACE, angiotensin-converting enzyme; AE, autoimmune encephalitis; ANA, antinuclear antibody; ASO, antistreptolysin O; CBC, complete blood count; CMP, comprehensive metabolic panel; CRP, C-reactive protein; CSF, cerebrospinal fluid; EEG, electroencephalogram; ESR, erythrocyte sedimentation rate; HHV, human herpes virus; HSV, herpes simplex virus; Ig, immunoglobulin; MRA, magnetic resonance angiography; VZV, varicella zoster virus; US, ultrasound.
  [a] There is an increased sensitivity when both serum and CSF AE panels ordered concurrently.

Anti-*N*-METHYL-ᴅ-ASPARTATE RECEPTOR ENCEPHALITIS
Epidemiology

Anti-NMDAR encephalitis accounts for 4% of all encephalitis cases, and is the leading cause of seropositive autoimmune encephalitis in children.[1,13,14] Initially described in adult females with ovarian teratomas, autoimmune encephalitis has subsequently been reported in men, women, and children with and without teratomas and in all age groups (youngest, 8 months old).[1,2,15] Approximately 40% of cases present under the age of 18 years.[16,17] Anti-NMDAR encephalitis occurs more frequently in girls and women (80%), except under the age of 12, where boys are slightly more likely to be affected.[1,14,15] Overall, about 40% of patients will have paraneoplastic disease, the overwhelming majority of which are women with ovarian teratomas.[1,2,14] About one-half of the women with anti-NMDAR encephalitis have a detectable neoplasm, with the age of greatest risk between 12 and 45 years of age. Testicular teratomas and small cell lung cancer have been reported in men; none have been under the age of 18 years.

Etiology

According to Dalmau and colleagues, the hypothesized inactivation of GABAergic neurons (which express higher NMDAR concentrations than other neuronal subtypes) may have a key role in the clinical presentation of NMDAR autoimmune encephalitis.[18] The disinhibition of the basal ganglia may also be associated with the psychomotor restlessness exhibited.[18] In general, the concepts of glutamate excitotoxicity and GABAergic dysfunction are believed to be central to the clinical phenotype commonly seen in anti-NMDAR encephalitis.[18]

Clinical Manifestations

In teenagers and adults, symptoms typically evolve in stages. A prodromal viral-like syndrome with fever and headache often occur first, followed by psychiatric symptoms that evolve over days to weeks.[1,14,19] Psychiatric symptoms and behavioral changes can be quite striking, including visual and auditory hallucinations, paranoia, anxiety, erratic or combative behavior, disinhibition, hypersexuality, catatonia, and severe insomnia.[11,14,17] These often lead to a misdiagnosis of a primary psychiatric disorder, such as schizophrenia or bipolar affective illness. Patients may later develop seizures, movement disorders (orolinguofacial dyskinesias, choreoathetoid movements, dystonic postures, muscle rigidity, or increased tone), impaired level of consciousness, autonomic instability, or hypoventilation.[20]

Children under the age of 12 years present differently, more commonly presenting with movement disorders and seizures as their initial symptoms.[9] Accompanying behavioral changes include agitation, aggression, tantrum behaviors, erratic sleep (insomnia mostly; less frequently, hypersomnia), as well as speech changes (decreased verbal output, mutism, perseveration, and echolalia).

Regardless of initial presentation, more than 90% of patients will have at least 3 of the following symptoms within 1 month of disease onset: psychiatric features, seizures, movement disorders, memory loss, changes in speech, decreased level of consciousness, autonomic instability, or hypoventilation.[14,15]

Diagnosis

Diagnosis is confirmed by detection of the NMDAR antibody in serum or CSF.[17] CSF is the gold standard, and is more sensitive than serum.[17–19] Serum NMDAR antibodies are detected concurrently in 85% of CSF seropositive cases.[17] Routine CSF studies are abnormal in about 80% of patients, revealing lymphocytic pleocytosis, elevated protein (often normal), or the presence of oligoclonal bands.[17–19] MRI may be abnormal in about one-third of children, with cortical and subcortical T2-weighted and fluid-attenuated inversion recovery abnormalities being seen, as well as leptomeningeal enhancement. The EEG may show a diffuse slowing of background activity.[17,20,21] Electrographic seizures seen during continuous EEG monitoring has been reported in 60% of cases.[20] Nonconvulsive status epilepticus has also been reported; as such, EEG (preferably 24-hour continuous EEG) is strongly recommended. Infectious, metabolic, paraneoplastic, toxic, and other autoimmune etiologies should be ruled out as part of the initial evaluation. MRI of the abdomen and pelvis is recommended for evaluation of neoplasm in female patients, and testicular ultrasound imaging for males.

LIMBIC ENCEPHALITIS

Limbic encephalitis (LE) describes a clinical syndrome characterized by inflammation in the limbic system resulting in subacute memory loss, seizures, and psychiatric symptoms. Refractory seizures may be a prominent feature. Several antineuronal antibodies have been associated with the clinical diagnosis of LE. Both glutamic acid decarboxylase 65 (GAD 65) and voltage-gaited potassium channel (VGKC) antibodies have been described in children.[6,22,23]

Voltage-Gaited Potassium Channel Encephalitis

VGKC antibody-mediated disease is considered to be a subtype of LE.[24,25] The clinical phenotype of VGKC encephalitis is better defined in adults with the recognition of the target proteins of LGI1 and CASPR2.[26] Children who test positive for VGKC antibodies do not have antibodies to the targets LGI1 or CASPR2.[23] There is speculation that the VGKC antibodies detected in the serum of children may be binding to intracellular domains and are not necessarily reflective of a pathologic mechanism. At this time, VGKC antibody positivity in children with an encephalopathy is thought to provide supporting evidence of autoimmune encephalitis, but it may reflect the presence of an inflammatory process as opposed to signifying a specific mechanism of disease.[23,24]

Glutamic Acid Decarboxylase Encephalitis

GAD 65 antibodies historically were believed to be directed toward intracellular proteins and, therefore, the symptoms were not thought to be directly from the antibody itself. In general, this syndrome is considered to be less responsive to immunotherapy as compared with subsets of autoimmune encephalitis in which the antibodies are targeting cell surface proteins. However, clinically, some patients with GAD 65–positive disease had marked improvements with immunotherapy and symptom severity changes that correlated with antibody titers. It is now hypothesized that there may be cell surface exposure during exocytosis. This potentially explains how GAD 65 antibodies seem to act more like classic paraneoplastic antibodies. At times, these antibodies are present without evidence of pathogenic properties, and in other cases their presence is accompanied by effects much like those found from antineuronal antibodies that target the cell surface.[22] VGKC-associated disease is felt to be more responsive to immunotherapy than GAD 65–related disease.[24]

Clinical manifestations

Children with LE present with prominent seizures along with short-term memory loss and a broad spectrum of psychiatric symptoms. Memory impairment is a key feature of LE, given the involvement of the hippocampus. The seizures characteristic of LE classically arise from the temporal lobes, but children with LE often have multifocal disease and many are refractory to antiepileptic medications. The classic facio–dystonic–brachial seizures seen in adults with VGKC antibodies have not been reported commonly in children. GAD 65 is also associated with insulin-dependent diabetes, as well as other autoimmune neurologic conditions, including stiff person syndrome and cerebellar ataxia. Therefore, a detailed neurologic examination can provide additional clues of an encephalopathy. Children rarely have associated oncologic disease, as compared with adults.

Diagnosis

There are no pediatric specific diagnostic criteria for LE. The adult criteria recently reported include the presence of:

1. Subacute onset of memory deficits, seizures, or psychiatric symptoms suggestive of limbic system involvement;
2. MRI demonstrating abnormalities on T2-weighted fluid-attenuated inversion recovery restricted to the medial temporal lobes;
3. CSF pleocytosis or EEG changes with epileptic or slow wave activity in the temporal lobes; and
4. No other reasonable diagnosis.[27,28]

   The investigators noted that a positive antineuronal antibody or abnormal PET scan also support the diagnosis.[6] MRI changes may occur later in the disease in some children with hippocampal atrophy despite the lack of initial changes on MRI.

HASHIMOTO'S ENCEPHALOPATHY
Epidemiology

Hashimoto's encephalopathy (HE) is a syndrome of neurologic and neuropsychiatric symptoms associated with increased levels of antithyroid antibodies in the absence of other etiologies such as infections, metabolic disease, and neoplasm. It is seen in both euthyroid and hypothyroid individuals, but only rarely in those with hyperthyroidism. The role of the antithyroid antibodies themselves are questioned, with the current understanding suggestive of the fact that they serve more as a markers of autoimmunity rather than directly acting on a common antigen in both thyroid and brain tissue.[29] Classically, patients with HE have a dramatic improvement with corticosteroids. This had led some to refer to this condition as "steroid-responsive encephalopathy associated with autoimmune thyroiditis." However, given that a significant number of cases do not have dramatic improvement with steroids alone and may require other medications, the inclusion of steroid responsiveness as a diagnostic criterion is questionable.

Clinical Manifestations

The clinical manifestations of HE are broad and can range from strokelike presentations to profound psychiatric disease. The most common symptom in children is seizures, but altered mental status, cognitive decline, psychosis, paranoia, hallucinations, focal neurologic defects, and movement disorders are also reported. Children can present with the sudden onset of seizures, agitation, or psychosis, or they can have a more relapsing–remitting course, manifesting as cognitive decline and psychiatric disease.

Diagnosis

The hallmark of this disease is elevated antithyroid antibodies. Recent diagnostic criteria have been proposed for adults including encephalopathy with seizures, hallucinations, or strokelike episodes, with either a normal MRI or nonspecific abnormalities, and positive thyroid antibodies. The adult criteria required subclinical or mild overt thyroid disease; however, many children with HE have normal thyroid function.[6] Both antithyroglobulin and antithyroid peroxidase serum antibodies have been found in patients with HE. CSF studies show a moderately elevated protein level in 60% of pediatric cases, but rarely any other abnormalities.[30,31] EEGs commonly show general or focal slowing without electrographic seizures, consistent with an encephalopathy. Computed tomography scans are usually normal, and although MRI is felt to be a more sensitive test for encephalitis, the majority (>70%) of children with a diagnosis of HE have normal imaging.[31] When abnormalities are seen, they have shown prolonged T2-weighted signals in subcortical white matter. Infectious, metabolic, paraneoplastic, toxic, and other autoimmune etiologies should be ruled out.

SERONEGATIVE AUTOIMMUNE ENCEPHALITIS

A subset of patients who phenotypically present as having a suspected autoimmune encephalitis will have negative antibody testing. Over the past few years there has been increased awareness of these "seronegative" patients for whom detection and diagnosis of autoimmune encephalitis is more challenging, but for whom rapid initiation of treatment is equally important.[16] As noted, the transition from "suspected" to "probable" autoimmune encephalitis is contingent on laboratory and/or imaging evidence of inflammation. Inadvertent delays in treatment often occur when syndrome recognition is impacted by the difficulty in the detection of autoantibodies.[14] Patients are routinely triaged to a provider for evaluation based on their initial presenting symptom(s). The detection and workup for the population of patients with autoimmune encephalitis seen first by a neurologist is often extensive.[24,32] However, for patients who present with primary psychiatric findings, the medical evaluation may be far more limited. As such, the number of patients with a potential autoimmune encephalitis that could be missed during the psychiatric triage process also increases exponentially. Regardless of the initial provider interface, psychiatry is routinely consulted to help in the management of the perceptual disturbances, catatonia, and behavioral agitation.

Other Forms of Autoimmune Encephalitis

Numerous other antibodies to neuronal proteins have been reported to cause autoimmune encephalitis, which can be separated into 2 broad categories: antibodies toward intracellular antigens and antibodies toward cell membrane or synaptic antigens (**Table 3**). In general, those with antibodies toward intracellular antigens are usually associated with neoplastic disease, and those with antibodies toward cell membrane or synaptic antigens are not. However, if any antibody is detected, screening for neoplasms is recommended. Detection of intracellular antigen antibodies has been associated with poor response to immunomodulatory therapy.

Although the majority of these antibodies have been reported in the adult population, more reports are increasing among the pediatric population. Many of them are associated with a clinical presentation of LE.

TREATMENT APPROACHES IN AUTOIMMUNE ENCEPHALITIS

There are 2 main goals in the treatment of autoimmune encephalitis: (1) decrease inflammation and (2) manage the symptoms of the disease to minimize ongoing injury.

Table 3	
Antibodies associated with autoimmune encephalitis	
Antibodies to Intracellular Antigens	**Antibodies to Cell Membrane or Synaptic Antigens**
Hu (ANNA-1)	NMDA receptor[a]
Ma2	Voltage-gaited potassium channel[a]
CV2	Leucine-rich glioma-inactivated 1
Collapsin response-mediator protein 5	Contactin-associated protein like 2
Antiphiphysin	AMPA receptor
Glutamic acid decarboxylase[a]	GABA B receptor
	Glycine receptor
	mGluR5 receptor

[a] Subtypes of autoimmune encephalitis seen in children.

Many patients require significant symptomatic management for the seizures, movement disorders, or psychiatric manifestations of the disease along with immunotherapy to maximize functionality and improve outcomes.

Immunotherapy

First-line immunotherapy includes intravenous (IV) steroids, IV immunoglobulin (IVIG), and plasmapheresis.[9,10] It is recommended that first-line therapy be initiated once a diagnosis of probable encephalitis is established, given the severity of autoimmune encephalitis. IV steroids are typically given as "pulse dosing" at 30 mg/kg up to 1000 mg. IV steroids are started for 3 to 5 consecutive days. Continued therapy with steroids varies and there are no clear treatment regimens. Some continue intermittent IV steroids anywhere from once a week to once a month, whereas others convert to daily steroids, either oral or IV, with doses in the 1 to 2 mg/kg/d range. It should be noted that systemic side effects are more frequently seen with oral steroids as opposed to intermittent IV steroid pulses. IVIG is typically given as 2 g/kg over 2 days, followed by dosing every 4 weeks. In some severe cases, IVIG is given more frequently, with the first 2 to 3 dosing cycles given every 2 weeks. The experience with plasmapheresis is variable. Some institutions prefer it as a first-line treatment and others reserve it for the more severely affected patients. Plasmapheresis is effective at removing peripheral antibodies, but there is question of how effective it is in removing CSF antibodies.[33–35] It should also be noted that plasmapheresis provides a short-term depletion of peripheral antibodies, and is unlikely to be effective as monotherapy for children with underlying autoimmune disease (autoimmune encephalitis). However, children with a postinfectious process may have sufficient benefit from plasmapheresis alone.

For children not showing improvement within 2 weeks, or declining on first-line therapy, escalating therapy to second-line treatments is recommended. Rituximab and cyclophosphamide are considered second-line agents, although cyclophosphamide is used less commonly in children than in adults.[9,10,36] In addition, oral agents such as mycophenolate mofetil or azathioprine may be useful for maintenance immunotherapy for children with a more protracted course.

There are few specific treatment recommendations for the various forms of autoimmune encephalitis. Antibodies to intracellular antigens such as GAD encephalitis may benefit from more intense immunotherapy at diagnosis because these antibodies are associated with a more destructive inflammatory process that can lead to extensive injury and permanent impairments. Formal consensus guidelines and treatment recommendations for NMDA encephalitis have not yet been defined. Some providers favor treating with rituximab at the time of diagnosis, because there is some evidence that this move may improve outcomes and decrease relapse rates. Others feel that, because many patients do well on first-line therapy alone, reserving a strong immunosuppressant treatment only for those with severe or protracted disease is warranted. Given that there are no trials in children with NMDA encephalitis currently available, optimal treatment remains an active question.[10]

HE is classically highly responsive to steroids. IV methylprednisolone is used most often, although oral prednisone is also reported. Given the high morbidity associated with high-dose daily oral steroids, IV methylprednisolone used every 2 to 4 weeks may be better tolerated.[19] Clinical improvement usually occurs in 1 to 10 days, although full recovery may take months. The average duration of treatment varies from 6 weeks to several years.[37] Approximately one-half of children with HE are not sufficiently responsive to steroids and require other immunomodulatory therapy. IVIG, rituximab, mycophenolate mofetil, and methotrexate have also been used.[37,38]

PATIENT OUTCOMES

Unfortunately, patient outcomes are highly variable ranging from full recovery to death.[6,38] According to Titulaer and colleagues, "most patients with anti-NMDAR encephalitis respond to immunotherapy" and "second line immunotherapy is usually effective when first-line treatments fail."[10] The time to recovery is variable. Some patients require 18 months or more to show recovery. More than one-half of patients diagnosed with NMDAR autoimmune encephalitis who were enrolled in the study authored by Titulaer and colleagues improved within the first 4 weeks when given first-line immunomodulatory therapies or undergoing tumor removal (if applicable).[10] The best prognostic indicators in this study were lack of a requirement for intensive care unit admission and having received prompt treatment.

MANAGEMENT OF PSYCHOSIS AND AGITATION IN AUTOIMMUNE ENCEPHALITIS

Autoimmune encephalitis places patients at risk for a broad range of psychiatric symptoms, including mood destabilization, behavioral changes, personality changes, confusion, disorientation, paranoia, hypervigilance, and hallucinatory phenomena.[39-42] The management of psychosis and agitation in these patients is frequently complicated by higher rates of autonomic instability and comorbid features of delirium and/or catatonia.[40,42] Patients with anti-NMDAR encephalitis in particular routinely present first with psychiatric chief complaints (approximately 75% of the time).[39,41] These patients often exhibit significant behavioral agitation and many have sensory perceptual disturbances.

Unfortunately, worsening of clinical status or symptom exacerbation with the use of antipsychotic medications is increasingly considered to be a potential feature of anti-NMDAR encephalitis.[41] However, this phenomenon may occur more broadly across the autoimmune encephalitis spectrum of illness. In general, the use of typical and atypical antipsychotics before the use of immunomodulatory agents may lead to symptom exacerbation, whereas the use of antipsychotics in conjunction with or after the administration of immunomodulatory agents (days to weeks) may be advantageous.

Patients with autoimmune encephalitis are believed to have higher risk stratification for neuroleptic malignant syndromes. Some patients have laboratory evidence of elevations in creatine kinase without (or premorbid to) the use of any antipsychotic medication regimen.[14] As a result, determining whether autonomic instability and rigidity are related to a neuroleptic malignant syndrome as compared with the natural disease trajectory of a patient with autoimmune encephalitis may be difficult.[14]

Patients with autoimmune encephalitis often respond well to the use of benzodiazepines (sometimes at escalating doses) for the management of agitation, particularly with the presentation of catatonia (**Table 4**). The use of olanzapine, quetiapine, risperidone, and haloperidol are routinely discussed as potential management options for symptoms of psychosis within case studies of patients diagnosed with autoimmune encephalitis.[17,31,39,41,42] However, little evidence is available to guide psychiatric treatment algorithms at this time.

Medications targeting insomnia as a presenting feature of delirium and agitation are also well-represented in case studies specific to autoimmune encephalitis. Treatments mentioned include diazepam, lorazepam, temazepam, alprazolam, zolpidem, mirtazapine, trazodone, clonidine, dexmedetomidine, propofol, gabapentin, and valproate.

MANAGEMENT OF DELIRIUM AND CATATONIA

At present, the majority of the literature available for the management of psychiatric symptoms in autoimmune encephalitis is in case report format. Many case reports specific to anti-NMDAR encephalitis discuss a period of psychomotor restlessness and altered sensorium that waxes and wanes, much like the traditional conceptualization of delirium[17,31,42] (**Table 5**). Although delirium is routinely treated with first- and second-generation antipsychotic medications, such medications are known to exacerbate catatonia. Conversely, although catatonia is treated effectively with the use of benzodiazepines, the use of benzodiazepines may propagate the cycle of delirium. As noted, medication choices in patients with autoimmune encephalitis may be further complicated by the presence of autonomic instability.[43–45]

The use of lorazepam and zolpidem within the field of catatonia research has given rise to the consideration of these agents for treating catatonic features associated with autoimmune encephalitis, sometimes with good success. Although the response to first- and second-generation antipsychotics alone may be suboptimal, many patients with autoimmune encephalitis are noted to respond well to lorazepam at escalating doses.[43–46] The pathophysiology and biochemical underpinnings of this phenomenon are not fully elucidated at present. Some theorize that the efficacy of lorazepam is more closely related to the phase of illness in which catatonic features are seen. Others theorize that the GABA modulation offered by lorazepam's mechanism of action leads to clinical improvement with or without features of catatonia.

Table 4 Features of catatonia	
Negativism	Doing the opposite action/behavior requested by the examiner
Mutism	Paucity or total lack of speech
Catalepsy	Fixed rigid postures independently initiated and held for prolonged period
Waxy flexibility	Fixed postures held by patient after being initiated by the examiner (ie, the patient is moved and then remains in this position)
Stupor	Lack of responsiveness, altered level of consciousness
Immobility	Lack of movement
Impulsivity	Intermittent excitement often with unpredictable and bizarre behaviors

Table 5 Features of delirium	
Psychomotor restlessness	Bicycling movements of lower extremities, swimming maneuvers of upper extremities, choreiform movements, stereotypies
Altered sensorium	Auditory and visual hallucinations, perceptual changes
Waxing and waning orientation	Confusion intermittently regarding person, time, place, and purpose
Insomnia	Interrupted sleep, day–night dysregulation, inability to sleep
Irritability and agitation	Difficulty to soothe, mood dysregulation, combative behaviors

It is important to note that the immunomodulatory therapies themselves often lead to pan symptom improvement or even full resolution of psychosis, agitation, catatonia, and delirium.[47–49]

MANAGEMENT OF RESIDUAL SYMPTOMS

Patients may present with residual symptoms of anxiety, inattention, impulsivity, psychosis, depression, obsessive–compulsive disorder, and panic in the postinflammatory phase of an autoimmune encephalitis.[44,48–50] For many families, the presence of residual symptoms is particularly distressing and they often struggle with grief reactions as they pursue the journey toward wellness with their child. Psychiatrists may be asked to help address these residual symptoms in concert with multidisciplinary treatment teams.[43,48] Usual treatment algorithms for anxiety, features of obsessive–compulsive disorder, panic, irritability, and depression may include selective serotonin reuptake inhibitors, serotonin and norepinephrine reuptake inhibitors, and tricyclic antidepressants. These agents may be efficacious in the postinflammatory phase and should be considered so long as there are no ongoing issues with autonomic instability. Likewise, the use of both typical and atypical antipsychotics is a reasonable strategy in treating residual symptoms of paranoia, auditory or visual hallucinations, delusional thought patterns, or mood lability leading to episodes of agitation. Patients who may have had very poor responses to psychotropic medication regimens during the active inflammation phase may find a new level of symptom relief and clinical efficacy with the use of these same medications in the postinflammatory phase (particularly when paired with ongoing immunomodulatory medication regimens).

One of the most important features of treating residual symptoms is the ongoing surveillance for potential flairs and relapse. Psychiatrists should work closely with multidisciplinary providers to include neurology, immunology, and rheumatology.[43,48] Understanding where the patient is at in their immunomodulatory treatment is often a key in determining next steps for residual symptoms (**Table 6**). As an example, a child may exhibit profound improvement immediately after infusions, but then have reemergence of symptoms as they approach their next monthly dose of IVIG or steroids. During this period, modifications in immunotherapy may be warranted to produce more sustained improvements. Rituximab is a common second-line agent in autoimmune encephalitis treatment. The clinical effects of B-cell depletion from rituximab may take 2 to 3 months to see. Some children receive just 1 course of rituximab, whereas others require sustained therapy with dosing every 6 months. Some children have improvements in cognitive domains (ie, language, calculation, logic, and memory) despite worsening behaviors or psychiatric symptoms during the recovery period.

Table 6
Child psychiatry appointment follow-up questions

Who is on your treatment team?	Neurology, rheumatology, immunology, primary care?
What is your current immunomodulatory regimen?	Intravenous steroids, oral steroids, B-cell modulatory agents, T-cell modulatory agents, plasmapheresis, intravenous immunoglobulin?
When was your last infusion or treatment?	Ask for specific dates and keep a log in clinic notes for follow-up pattern analysis
When is your next scheduled treatment?	Clarify timeline of symptoms before and after treatment if making any medication changes

Behavioral and psychiatric symptoms may also worsen as children meet increased demands, such as returning to school. It is important to determine if these changes are due to a flare of the encephalitis versus behavioral changes related to stressors. A flare of autoimmune encephalitis would include worsening in other domains such as cognition, language, and seizures in addition to the behavioral/psychiatric symptoms.

SUMMARY AND DISCUSSION

Autoimmune encephalitis has captured the attention of emergency room physicians, primary care providers, gynecologists, oncologists, psychiatrists, rheumatologists, immunologists, and neurologists alike. Fortunately, there is a growing body of literature now available on the topic of autoimmune encephalitis. However, there are few, if any, resources available that outline treatment algorithms for psychiatric care symptoms that clinicians encounter. Consensus is also needed in determining reasonable approaches to the workup, immunomodulatory regimens offered, and timelines for escalation of care. Child psychiatrists must become familiar with the diagnosis of autoimmune encephalitis given that they may be the first provider to evaluate patients with new onset neuropsychiatric symptoms. Given the complexity of this diagnostic spectrum, barriers in phenotype recognition are to be expected (**Box 1**). In general, if clinicians identify a patient who has acute onset psychiatric symptoms paired with seizures or focal neurologic findings, the suspicion for autoimmune encephalitis

Box 1
Barriers to pattern recognition in autoimmune encephalitis

- Potential for delay in diagnosis
- Difficulty in obtaining antibody panel testing outside of academic centers
- Difficulty in obtaining neuropsychological testing
- "Small" number of patients who fit diagnostic criteria annually (particularly in more remote locations)
- Confounding variables in terms of medication effects versus side effects during acute phase of illness
- Variation in immunomodulatory treatment approaches
- Many case reports but difficult to create multisite randomized controlled trials
- Difficulty navigating multidisciplinary treatment often required

should be raised. If there are additional elements such as a rapid decline, autonomic instability, cognitive dulling, neurologic deficits, or loss of functional skills, then psychiatrists must advocate for a full medical workup for their patient. Early recognition allows for prompt treatment, which is often a critical component to patient recovery and clinical outcomes.[49,50] Ongoing multisite and multispecialty collaborative efforts are required in moving forward with phenotype recognition and the creation of standard of care models for the autoimmune encephalitides.

REFERENCES

1. Dalmau J, Tüzün E, Wu HY, et al. Paraneoplastic anti-N-methyl-D aspartate receptor encephalitis associated with ovarian teratoma. Ann Neurol 2007;61(1): 25–36.
2. Leypoldt F, Wandinger K, Bien C, et al. Autoimmune encephalitis. Eur Neurol Rev 2013;8(1):31–7.
3. Kayser M, Dalmau J. The emerging link between autoimmune disorders and neuropsychiatric disease. J Neuropsychiatry Clin Neurosci 2011;23(1):90–7.
4. Van Mater H. Pediatric inflammatory brain diseases: a diagnostic approach. Curr Opin Rheumatol 2014;26(5):553–61.
5. Lancaster E. The diagnosis and treatment of autoimmune encephalitis. J Clin Neurol 2016;12(1):1–13.
6. Graus F, Titulaer MJ, Balu R, et al. A clinical approach to diagnosis of autoimmune encephalitis. Lancet Neurol 2016;15(4):391–404.
7. Gaspard N. Autoimmune epilepsy. Continuum 2016;22(1):227–45.
8. Lee SK, Lee ST. The laboratory diagnosis of autoimmune encephalitis. J Epilepsy Res 2016;6(2):45–52.
9. Dale R, Gorman M, Lim M. Autoimmune encephalitis in children: clinical phenomenology, therapeutics, and emerging challenges. Curr Opin Neurol 2017;30(3): 334–44.
10. Titulaer MJ, McCracken L, Gabilondo I, et al. Treatment and prognostic factors for long-term outcome in patients with anti-NMDA receptor encephalitis: an observational cohort study. Lancet Neurol 2013;12(2):157–65.
11. Hacohen Y, Wright S, Waters P, et al. Paediatric autoimmune encephalopathies: clinical features, laboratory investigations and outcomes in patients with or without antibodies to known central nervous system autoantigens. J Neurol Neurosurg Psychiatry 2013;84(7):748–55.
12. Albert D, Pluto CP, Weber A, et al. Utility of neurodiagnostic studies in the diagnosis of autoimmune encephalitis in children. Pediatr Neurol 2016;55:37–45.
13. Gable M, Sheriff H, Dalmau J, et al. The frequency of autoimmune N-methyl-D-aspartate receptor encephalitis surpasses that of individual viral etiologies in young individuals enrolled in the California Encephalitis Project. Clin Infect Dis 2012;54(7):899–904.
14. Armangue T, Petit-Pedrol M, Dalmau J. Autoimmune encephalitis in children. J Child Neurol 2012;27(11):1460–9.
15. Armangue T, Titulaer MJ, Málaga I, et al. Pediatric anti-N-methyl-D-aspartate receptor encephalitis-clinical analysis and novel findings in a series of 20 patients. J Pediatr 2013;162(4):850–6.
16. Lim M, Hacohen Y, Vincent A. Autoimmune encephalopathies. Pediatr Clin North Am 2015;62:667–85.
17. Dalmau J, Gleichman A, Hughes E, et al. Anti-NMDA-receptor-encephalitis: case series and analysis of the effects of antibodies. Lancet Neurol 2008;7:1091–8.

18. Dalmau J, Lancaster E, Martinez-Hernandez E, et al. Clinical experience and laboratory investigations in patients with anti-NMDAR encephalitis. Lancet Neurol 2011;10:63–74.
19. Pruss H, Dalmau J, Harm L, et al. Retrospective analysis of NMDA receptor antibodies in encephalitis of unknown origin. Neurology 2010;75:1735–9.
20. Wright S, Vincent A. Pediatric autoimmune epileptic encephalopathies. J Child Neurol 2017;32(4):418–28.
21. Florance N, Davis L, Lam C, et al. Anti-N-methyl-d-aspartate receptor (NMDAR) encephalitis in children and adolescents. Ann Neurol 2009;66:11–8.
22. Mishra N, Rodan L, Nita D, et al. Antiglutamic acid decarboxylase antibody associated limbic encephalitis in a child: expanding the spectrum of pediatric inflammatory brain diseases. J Child Neurol 2014;29(5):677–83.
23. Hacohen Y, Singh R, Rossi M, et al. Clinical relevance of voltage-gated potassium channel-complex antibodies in children. Neurology 2015;85(11):967–75.
24. Wagner J, Schoene-Bake J, Witt J, et al. Distinct white matter integrity in glutamic acid decarboxylase and voltage-gated potassium channel-complex antibody-associated limbic encephalitis. Epilepsia 2016;57(3):475–83.
25. Newey CR, Sarwal A. Hyponatremia and voltage gated potassium channel antibody associated limbic encephalitis. J Neurol Neurophysiol 2014;5(2):195.
26. Suleiman J, Brilot F, Lang B, et al. Autoimmune epilepsy in children: case series and proposed guidelines for identification. Epilepsia 2013;54(6):1036–45.
27. Gultekin S, Rosenfeld M, Voltz R, et al. Paraneoplastic limbic encephalitis: neurological symptoms, immunological findings and tumour association in 50 patients. Brain 2000;123(Pt 7):1481–94.
28. Graus F, Saiz A. Limbic encephalitis: a probably under-recognized syndrome. Neurologia 2005;20(1):24–30.
29. Zhou J, Xu B, Lopes J, et al. Hashimoto encephalopathy: literature review. Acta Neurol Scand 2017;135(3):285–90.
30. Laurent C, Capron J, Quillerou B, et al. Steroid-responsive encephalopathy associated with autoimmune thyroiditis (SREAT): characteristics, treatment and outcome in 251 cases from the literature. Autoimmun Rev 2016;15(12):1129–33.
31. Brenton J, Goodkin H. Antibody-mediated autoimmune encephalitis in childhood. Pediatr Neurol 2016;60:13–23.
32. Wright S, Hacohen Y, Jacobson L, et al. N-methyl-D-aspartate receptor antibody-mediated neurological disease: results of a UK-based surveillance study in children. Arch Dis Child 2015;100(6):521–6.
33. Furneaux H, Reich L, Posner J. Autoantibody synthesis in the central nervous system of patients with paraneoplastic syndromes. Neurology 1990;40(7):1085–91.
34. Gresa-Arribas N, Titulaer M, Torrents A, et al. Antibody titres at diagnosis and during follow-up of anti-NMDA receptor encephalitis: a retrospective study. Lancet Neurol 2014;13:167–77.
35. Graus F, Abos J, Roquer J, et al. Effect of plasmapheresis on serum and CSF autoantibody levels in CNS paraneoplastic syndromes. Neurology 1990;40(10):1621–3.
36. Dale RC, Brilot F, Duffy LV, et al. Utility and safety of rituximab in pediatric autoimmune and inflammatory CNS disease. Neurology 2014;83(2):142–50.
37. Kirshner H. Hashimoto's encephalopathy: a brief review. Curr Neurol Neurosci Rep 2014;14(9):476.
38. Quek A, Britton J, McKeon A, et al. Autoimmune epilepsy: clinical characteristics and response to immunotherapy. Arch Neurol 2012;69(5):582–93.

39. Schumacher L, Mann A, MacKenzie J. Agitation management in pediatric males with anti-N-methyl-D-aspartate receptor encephalitis. J Child Adolesc Psychopharmacol 2016;26(10):939–43.
40. Ryan S, Costello D, Cassidy E, et al. Anti-NMDA receptor encephalitis: a cause of acute psychosis and catatonia. J Psychiatr Pract 2013;19(2):157–61.
41. Maneta E, Garcia G. Psychiatric manifestations of anti NMDA receptor encephalitis: neurobiological underpinnings and differential diagnostic implications. Psychosomatics 2013;55(1):37–44.
42. Granerod J, Ambrose H, Davies N, et al, UK Health Protection Agency (HPA) Aetiology of Encephalitis Study Group. Causes of encephalitis and differences in their clinical presentations in England: a multicentre, population-based prospective study. Lancet Infect Dis 2010;10(12):835–44.
43. Mann A, Machado N, Liu N, et al. A multidisciplinary approach to the treatment of anti-NMDA receptor antibody encephalitis: a case and review of the literature. J Neuropsychiatry Clin Neurosci 2012;24:247–54.
44. Barry H, Hardiman O, Healy D, et al. Anti-NMDA receptor encephalitis: an important differential diagnosis in psychosis. Br J Psychiatry 2011;199:508–9.
45. Kuo Y, Tsai H, Lai M, et al. Anti-NMDA receptor encephalitis with the initial presentation of psychotic mania. J Clin Neurosci 2012;19:896–8.
46. Day B, Eisenman L, Black J, et al. A case study of voltage gated potassium channel antibody related limbic encephalitis with PET/MRI findings. Epilepsy Behav Case Rep 2015;4:23–6.
47. Merchut MP. Management of voltage gated potassium channel antibody disorders. Neurol Clin 2010;23(4):941–59.
48. Brenton J, Kim J, Schwarz R. Approach to the management of pediatric onset anti-N-methyl-D-aspartate receptor encephalitis: a case series. J Child Neurol 2016;31(9):1150–5.
49. Byrne S, Walsh C, Hacohen Y, et al. Earlier treatment of NMDAR antibody encephalitis in children results in better outcome. Neurol Neuroimmunol Neuroinflamm 2015;2(4):e130.
50. Pillai SC, Hacohen Y, Tantsis E, et al. Infectious and autoantibody-associated encephalitis: clinical features and long term outcome. Pediatrics 2015;135(4):e974–84.

Pediatric Psychogenic Nonepileptic Seizures
A Concise Review

Julia L. Doss, PsyD[a],*, Sigita Plioplys, MD[b]

KEYWORDS

- Psychogenic nonepileptic seizures • Conversion • Functional neurologic disorder
- Epilepsy • Pediatric

KEY POINTS

- Psychogenic nonepileptic seizures in youth is a complex biopsychosocial disorder with high rates of medical and psychiatric comorbidities.
- Timely recognition and effective treatment of psychogenic nonepileptic seizures in youth requires a team approach, with both medical and mental health professionals conducting comprehensive evaluations and providing diagnostic feedback and interdisciplinary treatment.
- Risk factors for psychogenic nonepileptic seizures in youth are different than in adults and include social and family stress, high rates of comorbid general medical and psychiatric diagnoses, and lifetime adversities, including violence and sexual abuse, but the rates are much lower than reported in adults with psychogenic nonepileptic seizures.
- Treatment entails both short-term symptom management and return to normal daily function and long-term treatment of psychiatric comorbidities.

INTRODUCTION

Psychogenic nonepileptic seizures (PNES) is a conversion disorder (Functional Neurologic Symptom Disorder in Diagnostic and Statistical Manual of Mental Disorders 5 [DSM 5])[1] involving alterations in behavior, motor activity, consciousness and sensation that resemble epileptic seizures.[2] Unlike epilepsy, PNES are not associated with epileptiform activity in the brain as measured with electroencephalography,[3] but seizurelike symptoms develop in response to psychological stress.[4] A conceptual biopsychosocial model of conversion proposes that unresolved psychological stress

Disclosure Statement: The authors have no disclosures.
[a] Department of Psychology, Minnesota Epilepsy Group, 225 Smith Avenue North, Suite 201, St Paul, MN 55102, USA; [b] Department of Child and Adolescent Psychiatry, Pediatric Neuropsychiatry Clinic, Ann and Robert H. Lurie Children's Hospital of Chicago, Northwestern University, 225 East Chicago Avenue, Box 10, Chicago, IL 60611, USA
* Corresponding author.
E-mail address: jdoss@mnepilepsy.net

Child Adolesc Psychiatric Clin N Am 27 (2018) 53–61
http://dx.doi.org/10.1016/j.chc.2017.08.007

childpsych.theclinics.com

creates a cascade effect of physical, emotional, and social consequences that perpetuate the physical symptoms.[5,6]

PNES represents up to 25% of all admissions to inpatient epilepsy monitoring units.[3,7,8] There are no population-based studies of PNES, but it is estimated that there are between 300,000 to 400,000 individuals with this condition in the United States alone.[2] Although this might be less common in the pediatric population than in adults, it is difficult to estimate its prevalence, as most studies of PNES originate from epilepsy centers in which video-electroencephalography (VEEG) aides in the most accurate diagnosis. Therefore, estimates of PNES prevalence from those studies are likely underrepresentative of the prevalence in the general population, where VEEG is less accessible.[9]

PNES in children is an understudied condition with severe medical and psychiatric comorbidity,[10–12] significant health care service burden,[13] and parental financial hardship because of missed work and cost of medical investigations.[7,14] Children with PNES who get incorrectly diagnosed with epilepsy receive unnecessary medical interventions and diagnostic tests, including intubation in the case of presumed status epilepticus. They experience academic and social difficulties because of frequent PNES episodes, missed school days, and cognitive and psychiatric side effects from the antiepileptic drugs (AEDs) given to treat their "seizures."[7,14]

Diagnostic delay in children ranges from weeks up to 3.5 years on average.[8] This delay is thought to be caused by multiple factors with the most common being misdiagnosis of epilepsy, lack of resources and access to VEEG, or family and patient not accepting that the child's symptoms have a psychological rather than physical origin.[2,15] Misdiagnosis can contribute to significant delay in treatment of underlying psychopathology, which may hamper PNES prognosis for remission in symptoms.[7] Several studies speculate that longer duration from onset of PNES symptoms to treatment can significantly impact response to the therapy, with higher rates of recidivism of symptoms and emergence of other somatic complaints.[16–18]

Psychogenic Nonepileptic Seizures Risk Factors

Historically, PNES was thought to occur as the result of a devastating experience, often sexual abuse.[3] Contrary to adults, this has not borne out in pediatric studies. In the risk factors study by Plioplys and colleagues,[19] youth with PNES were found to have a complex profile of interrelated biopsychosocial risk factors. Compared with their siblings, the youth with PNES had significantly more lifetime comorbid general medical, neurologic (including epilepsy) and psychiatric diagnoses; used more medications and intensive medical services; experienced greater anxiety sensitivity; and used more venting (solitary emotional expression) coping. The patients also reported significantly more lifetime adversities than their siblings.

In the study by Plioplys and colleagues,[19] individual child-related factors, such as fearful response to physical sensations, bullying, learning struggles, and high frequency of comorbid internalizing psychiatric disorders, made the youth more vulnerable to the development of PNES. In an earlier study examining children with epilepsy (CWE) and those with PNES, anxiety sensitivity (ie, fearful perception of somatic symptoms when anxious) was found to be more common in the youth with PNES than in those with CWE.[20]

Family functioning is postulated as impacting the development of PNES, but few studies examine this risk factor in children with PNES specifically. Youth with PNES report family stress as a significant daily hassle, although this stress was not significantly different from that reported by their siblings.[19] Family modeling and learned behavior theories postulate that youth can develop conversion/functional symptoms from witnessing maladaptive response to illness in family members or being reinforced for illness behaviors in themselves.[21–23] In a pilot study of assessment tools for pediatric PNES, Salpekar and colleagues[20] found that parents of PNES children, compared with parents of CWE only, reported higher somatization scores in themselves and more somatic symptoms in their children. Thus, greater awareness of and focus on somatic complaints in the parents may have a role in the development of the psychosomatic symptoms in their children.[6] Plioplys and colleagues[24] also found that parents perceived greater medical vulnerability in their children with PNES than those without PNES. This too could lead parents to place greater focus on somatic symptoms in children, inadvertently reinforcing the psychosomatic symptoms as they develop.[6]

Parental psychopathology is a well-known risk factor for mental disorders, including conversion, in children.[25–27] Salpekar and colleagues[20] found significantly higher Beck Depression Inventory scores[28] and a trend for higher Beck Anxiety Inventory scores[29] in mothers of children with PNES compared with mothers of CWE. The few studies of psychopathology in parents of children with other somatic conditions found that parents endorse more symptoms of anxiety, depression, and somatization than parents of normal controls.[22,25] A study of adults with PNES also found higher rates of psychopathology in the family members. In this study, subjects also perceived family members as less interested in their activities and values, reported poor communication between family members, and reported higher rates of family conflict compared with a control group of patients with epilepsy.[30]

Assessment and Diagnosis

A detailed history is critical in the early PNES evaluation phase, whether the patient presents first to a pediatrician or to a neurologist. Necessary information to gather includes age of onset, semiology of events, and similarity between the events of interest.[31] The differential diagnosis between physiologic nonepileptic events, such as complex tics, syncope, complex migraine headaches, sleep disorders, and PNES, must include a thorough history, physical and neurologic examination, and VEEG capturing the paroxysmal event without an ictal electroencephalography (EEG) epileptiform correlate. Additional testing such as ictal prolactin, heart variability, oximetry, cognitive and psychological functioning, sleep study, and brain MRI can be used as supplemental data, but they are not diagnostic for PNES.

Differential diagnosis between PNES and epileptic seizures can be complex, as there are no specific clinical signs and symptoms distinguishing these 2 disorders. Also, a positive neurologic history (comorbid epilepsy, history of traumatic brain injury) can be found in almost half of children with PNES, and a positive family history of epilepsy was present in 35% of children with PNES.[8] Presence of EEG abnormalities in patients with PNES does not necessarily confirm diagnosis of epilepsy, because normal EEG variants can be misinterpreted as interictal epileptiform discharges in patients without epilepsy.

Three clinical criteria yield a positive diagnostic predictive value of 85% in patients with PNES. The criteria are (1) at least 2 PNES episodes per week, (2) refractory to at least 2 AEDs, and (3) at least 2 routine EEGs without epileptiform activity despite ongoing seizurelike episodes. Using "the rule of 2s" documenting seizure frequency, EEG abnormalities, and drug treatment response before VEEG may help with definitive diagnosis of PNES.[31] Therefore, pediatric patients who present with multiple varied paroxysmal episodes, who have refractory seizures despite multiple medication trials, or those who have had negative EEGs findings during the typical episodes should be evaluated for PNES.[32]

Psychiatric assessment is an essential part of the PNES evaluation. DSM 5 criteria[1] outline key criteria of conversion disorder that aid in the diagnosis and treatment. Ideally, psychiatric evaluation occurs at the same time as the neurologic assessment, because it provides information about the underlying stressors and emotional factors contributing to the patient's symptoms in question.[12] Patients are frequently unaware of their distress or unable to understand the link between stressors and their symptoms; thus, psychiatric evaluation aides in delivery of the PNES diagnosis and establishes a basis for psychological treatment.[33,34]

Gates[3] proposed a method for providing diagnostic feedback in the context of the epilepsy evaluation involving an integrated, interdisciplinary presentation by the neurologist and the mental health provider. Feedback to patients and their families involves a thorough review of the interdisciplinary diagnostic process and discussion about the objective findings and their meaningful interpretation, providing clear explanation why the patient's condition is not epileptic. The use of a team approach is described in multiple reports, with the neurologist describing the medical evaluation and negative EEG and the mental health professional describing how emotional distress can manifest as seizurelike symptoms.[3,12,33] Youth, unlike adults with PNES, have parents or caregivers present during their evaluations. Diagnostic feedback be provided to parents and children separately at first to effectively address parent's questions and potentially negative reactions before presenting it to the children.[12,34,35] This method may help alleviate concerns and mitigate initial resistance to the PNES diagnosis. This method also allows the clinicians to frame a conceptualization of the problem with the parents and emphasize that this diagnosis does not indicate that the child is "faking".[12] Reuber[15] noted that nearly all patients have some initial resistance or disbelief about the PNES diagnosis. Communication of this diagnosis to patients and families may require multiple sessions. A significant number of patients with PNES seek more than one opinion about their diagnosis, demonstrating lack of understanding, acceptance, or both, which can contribute to treatment delay.[7,15]

Comorbidities

Youth with PNES have high rates of co-occurring medical and psychiatric disorders. They more often seek medical care in the emergency department (6.1 vs 2 times compared with siblings), experience other types of somatic complaints, and report more physical illnesses than the same-age siblings.[19] Epilepsy is the most commonly co-occurring neurologic disorder present in about one-third of patients with PNES.[8,19]

Comorbid psychopathology is reported in 16% to 100% of youth with PNES.[8,19,33–37] It is more frequent and severe in adolescents with PNES than in children younger than 13 years (48.6% vs 16%).[8] Youth with PNES have more severe and prevalent comorbid psychopathology, such as internalizing disorders, posttraumatic stress disorder (PTSD), anxiety sensitivity (identification of body sensations as dangerous), and somatization than their siblings.[19] Regarding specific psychiatric diagnoses, significantly more youth with PNES than siblings had anxiety (83.6% vs 34.3%; $F[1,33] = 18.6$; $P<.0001$), depression (43.6% vs 14.3%; $F[1,33] = 5.1$; $P = .03$), and PTSD diagnoses (25.5% vs 2.9%; $F[1,33] = 5.8$; $P = .02$).[19] Multiple psychiatric disorders are typically present although may be undiagnosed at the time of presentation for evaluation of PNES.[18,19,38] Pediatric PNES is not a separate diagnosis but typically is diagnosed under the DSM 5 as a conversion disorder.[1] Prior classifications placed some forms of PNES under dissociative disorders, which are endorsed in adult PNES studies,[39] but this was not found in the PNES youth prospective study.[19]

School difficulties, including learning problems, bullying, social phobia, and school refusal are significant risk factors for PNES in youth.[19,40] Pediatric patients with PNES either do not recognize or do not communicate struggles associated with school to their parents or physicians. In a recent study by Doss and colleagues,[40] 60% of patients with PNES reported learning problems; only 13% of parents recognized those struggles. In this study, youth with PNES had normal IQs but reported more school struggles than siblings, with factors like bullying, anxiety, and subtle language problems contributing to their reported learning problems. They also missed more days of school (7.1 vs 1.7) compared with siblings.

Treatment

Treatment for children with PNES should not only entail management of PNES symptoms, but also the comorbid psychopathology.[19] There are no known PNES treatment studies involving children that prospectively assessed outcome of treatment. Several studies have reviewed PNES treatment in children and found that 55% to 80% of the subjects have cessation in PNES symptoms after several treatment sessions.[18,41,42]

Barriers to treatment include misdiagnosis, difficulty communicating the PNES diagnosis to patients and their family members, and various levels of acceptance of this diagnosis ranging from full acceptance to full denial.[43] A multidisciplinary approach is thought to be the most efficacious treatment approach.[3,12,33] The diagnosing neurologist or primary care physician must remain involved in the clinical care of the patient with PNES to continue to assure the family on the accuracy of the diagnosis, taper off and discontinue AEDs when indicated, and respond to questions about the ongoing or new medical symptoms. The mental health treatment team, comprising a psychiatrist and a psychologist or other mental health therapist, then addresses the management of PNES symptoms and underlying stressors responsible for the conversion disorder and addresses comorbid psychopathology.[33,34] Because of the lack of training and experience with conversion disorder, few psychiatrists and psychologists feel competent to treat this disorder, resulting in one of the most significant barriers to successful treatment.[34,35]

The psychiatric treatment of conversion disorder is based on a combination of multimodal individual and family therapy, along with appropriate educational and social interventions. There is no evidence that AEDs or psychopharmacologic agents, specifically antidepressants or antianxiety medications, are effective in the treatment of conversion disorder in youth. Cognitive behavior treatment, family therapy, and psychodynamic/interpersonal therapies are all postulated to treat PNES in adults,[2,43] but such studies are not available in children with PNES. Retrospective studies using a combination of these methods found significant improvement in PNES symptoms in youth within the first 3 months of therapy.[18,40] Little is known about long-term prognosis or functioning after treatment in youth or adults with PNES.[10,44]

Treatment of PNES is complex and requires both short- and long-term treatment goals.[34,35] Creating a response plan for parents and teachers is recommended.[35] Caplan and colleagues[35] provides a framework for the initial management of the PNES symptoms and the underlying emotional processes that caused the conversion symptoms. Individual treatment with the child and separate parenting sessions are recommended within this framework. Therapeutic work with the parent initially involves explaining that the child's symptoms are not fake or intentionally driven by the child. Instead, parents are educated about how underlying emotions can propagate involuntary physical symptoms. In addition, it is explained to parents that these outwardly alarming episodes are medically safe and that patients with PNES tend to used self-protective mechanisms (consciously or subconsciously). Parents are encouraged to follow a response plan during these events to allow them to respond to these episodes calmly and in ways that do not accidentally reinforce PNES symptoms. Additionally, coaching parents to respond to their child both empathically and with expectations about gradual increases in daily functioning, helps to promote symptom improvement over time. Goals for individual work with the child initially entail reduction in PNES physical symptoms or in the impact of these symptoms on functioning, return to normal daily activities, and effective management of stressors,[45] After the child develops some coping skills, and the physical symptoms are better controlled, work begins with the child to help them gain insight into the triggers for underlying emotional distress.[35] Comorbid school, learning, and peer struggles should be addressed early in treatment to enhance functioning and promote positive coping.

Long-term treatment of conversion disorder and the underlying psychopathologic conditions may also be necessary. Although there are no studies of long-term outcomes of youth with PNES, high rates of new somatic symptoms, worsening comorbid psychopathology, and poor long-term functioning are reported in studies of other forms of conversion disorder, especially when the underlying psychopathologic condition is not treated.[22,23]

Most patients can be treated in an outpatient treatment setting with a combination of therapy and psychotropic medication to both treat the symptoms of conversion disorder and the comorbid psychopathology. Psychiatric treatment of comorbid psychiatric disorders uses standard evidence-based psychopharmacologic and psychotherapeutic modalities along with appropriate educational and family interventions.

There are circumstances in which the child with PNES may need intensive psychiatric services. Caplan and colleagues[35] indicated the following criteria may warrant recommendations for inpatient admission: uncontrolled, daily PNES episodes present at school and home; PNES continuing for longer than 1 year and school absence longer than 3 months; severe PTSD, mood disorders, or psychosis; suicidal thoughts, plans, or attempts; and recently revealed history of abuse or unsafe home environment. Partial hospitalization programs may also be used if the above criteria are present but less severe, the child has been out of school for a significant period (3 months or more) and reintegration to school or home is unsuccessful, or if there is open resistance from the child or the parents to implement behavioral treatment strategies to control the symptoms. A limited number of specialized, combined medical and psychiatric inpatient and partial hospital programs have been developed in the United States to specifically treat patients with PNES and other somatic symptom-related disorders, and additional programs are in early stages of development. Such programs should be considered when regional or outpatient programs are not available or cannot meet the high level of integrated collaboration among health care providers that PNES patients may require.

Medical/rehabilitation treatments, such as physical therapy for other comorbid physical symptoms such as gait abnormalities, abnormal movements, or muscle weakness, and occupational therapy for fine motor or daily care issues, can be included in conjunction with any level of care (inpatient psychiatric, partial hospital, and outpatient psychotherapy). Inclusion of these rehabilitation treatment modalities is considered standard of care in the combined medical/psychiatric treatment programs noted above. Medical rehabilitation facilities (without intensive psychiatric treatment embedded therein) treat a variety of other forms of conversion disorder with a focus on mind-body associations and return to functioning. These facilities are most suited for those patients and families who resist accepting that PNES is a psychological disorder and desire to focus more exclusively on return to function.[12,35] It should be noted, however, that patients undergoing more purely physical treatment without intensive psychiatric services may struggle to make the necessary treatment gains that facilitate the full return to daily functioning, and may also experience re-emergence of conversion symptoms during future periods of increased emotional distress.

Prognosis is postulated to be better in children than in adults,[17] with PNES and symptom improvement expected to be quicker. This finding is especially true if diagnosis occurs close to the time of initiation of conversion symptoms, highlighting a significance of early recognition and diagnosis of PNES.[7,10]

SUMMARY

PNES is a complicated biopsychosocial disorder with significant morbidity; high cost in children's social, emotional, family, and academic functioning; and health care service utilization. Misdiagnosis and diagnostic delay, resulting from both lack of access to approved standards for diagnosing and service providers comfortable with diagnosing and treating this disorder, impact prognosis. Treatment shortly after symptom onset is thought to provide the best chance for remission.

REFERENCES

1. American Psychiatric Association. Diagnostic and statistical manual of mental disorders (5th edition). Washington, DC: American Psychiatric Publishing; 2013.
2. LaFrance WC Jr, Baker GA, Duncan R, et al. Minimum requirements for the diagnosis of psychogenic nonepileptic seizures: a staged approach: a report from the International League against Epilepsy Nonepileptic Seizures Task Force. Epilepsia 2013;54(11):2005–18.
3. Gates J. Nonepileptic seizures: time for progress. Epilepsy Behav 2000;1:2–6.
4. Reuber M, House A, Pukrop R, et al. Somatization, dissociation and general psychopathology in patients with psychogenic non-epileptic seizures. Epilepsy Res 2003;57:159–67.
5. Baslet G. Psychogenic non-epileptic seizures: a model of their pathogenic mechanism. Seizure 2011;20(1):1–13.
6. Brown R, Reuber M. Towards an integrative theory of psychogenic non-epileptic seizures (PNES). Clin Psychol Rev 2016;47:55–70.
7. Valente K, Alessi R, Vincentiis S, et al. Risk factors for diagnostic delay in psychogenic non-epileptic seizures among children and adolescents. Neurology 2017;67:71–7.
8. Patel H, Scott E, Dunn D, et al. Non-epileptic seizures in children. Epilepsia 2007;48:2086–92.
9. Reuber M. Psychogenic nonepileptic seizures: answers and questions. Epilepsy Behav 2008;12(4):622–35.
10. Lancman ME, Asconape JJ, Graves S, et al. Psychogenic seizures in children: long-term analysis of 43 cases. J Child Neurol 1994;9:404–7.
11. Plioplys S. Children with psychogenic non-epileptic seizures: high incidence of comorbid medical illnesses. Scientific proceedings of the AACAP, San Diego (CA), chapter 207. vol. XXXIII. 2006. p. 234.
12. Plioplys S, Asato M, Bursch B, et al. Multidisciplinary management of pediatric nonepileptic seizures. J Am Acad Child Adolesc Psychiatry 2007;46:1491–5.
13. Ahmedani B, Osborne J, Nerenz D, et al. Diagnosis, costs and utilization for non-epileptic seizures in a US healthcare setting. Psychosomatics 2013;54:28–34.
14. Reilly C, Menlove L, Fenton V, et al. Psychogenic nonepileptic seizures in children: a review. Epilepsia 2013;54(10):1715–24.

15. Reuber M. Communicating the diagnosis. In: Dworetzky B, Baslet G, editors. Psychogenic nonepileptic seizures: toward the integration of care. New York: Oxford University Press; 2017. p. 179–92.

16. Wyllie E, Glazer J, Benbadis S, et al. Psychiatric features of children and adolescents with pseudoseizures. Arch Pediatr Adolesc Med 1999;153:244–8.

17. Gudmundsson O, Prendergast M, Foreman D, et al. Outcome of pseudoseizures in children and adolescents: a 6 year symptom survival analysis. Dev Med Child Neurol 2001;43:547–51.

18. Doss J, & Palmquist M. Treatment of psychogenic non-epileptic seizures in the pediatric population. Annual Meeting of the American Epilepsy Society. Seattle, December 5-9, 2014.

19. Plioplys S, Doss J, Siddarth P, et al. A multi-site controlled study of risk factors for pediatric psychogenic non-epileptic seizures. Epilepsia 2014;55(11):1739–47.

20. Salpekar JA, Plioplys S, Siddarth P, et al. Pediatric psychogenic nonepileptic seizures: a study of assessment tools. Epilepsy Behav 2010;17:50–5.

21. Goodman JE, McGrath PJ. Mothers' modeling influences children's pain during a cold pressor task. Pain 2003;104:559–65.

22. Kashikar-Zuck S, Lynch AM, Slater S, et al. Family factors, emotional functioning, and functional impairment in juvenile fibromyalgia syndrome. Arthritis Rheum 2008;59:1392–8.

23. Walker LS, Garber J, Greene JW. Somatization symptoms in pediatric abdominal pain patients: relation to chronicity of abdominal pains and parent somatization. J Abnorm Child Psychol 1991;19:379–94.

24. Plioplys S, Doss J, Siddarth P, et al. Risk factors for pediatric non-epileptic seizures (NES): Psychiatric and medical comorbidities. Annual Meeting of American Epilepsy Society. San Diego, December 1-5, 2012.

25. Garber J, Zeman J, Walker LS. Recurrent abdominal pain in children: psychiatric diagnoses and parental psychopathology. J Am Acad Child Adolesc Psychiatry 1990;2:648–56.

26. Hodges K, Kline JJ, Barbero G, et al. Depressive symptoms in children with recurrent abdominal pain and in their families. J Pediatr 1985;107:622–6.

27. Hodges K, Kline JJ, Barbero G, et al. Anxiety in children with recurrent abdominal pain and their parents. Psychosomatics 1985;26(859):862–6.

28. Beck AT, Ward CH, Mendelson M, et al. An inventory for measuring depression. Arch Gen Psychiatry 1961;4:561–71.

29. Beck AT, Steer RA. Beck anxiety inventory manual. San Antonio (TX): Harcourt Brace and Company; 1993.

30. Krawetz P, Fleisher W, Pillay N, et al. Family functioning in subjects with pseudoseizures and epilepsy. J Nerv Ment Dis 2001;189:38–43.

31. Davis BJ. Predicting nonepileptic seizures utilizing seizure frequency, EEG, and response to medication. Eur Neurol 2004;51:153–6.

32. Rathod J, Benbadis S. Diagnostic challenges for the neurologist. In: Dworetzky B, Baslet G, editors. Psychogenic nonepileptic seizures: toward the integration of care. New York: Oxford University Press; 2017. p. 266–78.

33. Caplan R, Plioplys S. Psychiatric features and management of children with psychogenic nonepileptic seizures. In: Schachter SC, LaFrance WC, editors. Gates and Rowan's nonepileptic seizures. Cambridge (UK): Cambridge University Press; 2010. p. 163–78.

34. Doss J, Robbins J. The roles of the patient and family. In: Dworetzky B, Baslet G, editors. Psychogenic nonepileptic seizures: toward the integration of care. New York: Oxford University Press; 2017. p. 266–78.

35. Caplan R, Doss J, Plioplys S, et al. Pediatric psychogenic non-epileptic seizures: a treatment guide. Switzerland: Springer International Publishing; 2017.
36. Vincentiis S, Valente KD, Thomé-Souza S, et al. Risk factors for psychogenic non-epileptic seizures in children and adolescents with epilepsy. Epilepsy Behav 2006;8:294–8.
37. Plioplys S, Doss J, Siddarth P, et al. Risk factors for comorbid psychopathology in youth with psychogenic nonepileptic seizures. Seizure 2016;38:32–7.
38. Plioplys S, Szwed S, Varn M. Psychiatric problems in children with psychogenic nonepileptic seizures (NES). Epilepsia 2005;46:159.
39. Akyuz G, Kugu N, Akyuz A, et al. Dissociation and childhood abuse history in epileptic and pseudoseizure patients. Epileptic Disord 2004;6:187–92.
40. Doss J, Caplan R, Siddarth P, et al. Risk factors for learning problems in youth with psychogenic non-epileptic seizures. Epilepsy Behav 2017;70(Pt A):135–9.
41. Sawchuck T, Buchhalter J. Psychogenic nonepilepic seizures in children: psychological presentation, treatment and short-term outcomes. Epilepsy Behav 2015;52:49–56.
42. Alper K. Nonepiletpic seizures. Neurologic Clinics 1994;12:153–73.
43. Myers L, Mathur V, Lancman M. Prolonged exposure therapy for the treatment of patients diagnosed with psychogenic non-epileptic seizurs (PNES) and post-traumatic stress disorder (PTSD). Epilepsy Behav 2017;66:86–92.
44. Bhatia MS, Sapra MA. Pseudoseizures in children: a profile of fifty cases. Clin Pediatr 2005;44:617–21.
45. Irwin K, Edwards M, Robinson R. Psychogenic non-epileptic seizures: management and prognosis. Arch Dis Child 2000;82:474–8.

A Review of the Prevention and Medical Management of Childhood Obesity

Kristin L. Anderson, MD

KEYWORDS

- Childhood obesity • Prevention plus • Motivational interviewing
- Cardiometabolic risks • Metformin • Behavioral interventions

KEY POINTS

- Revised classification will include higher degrees of obesity that are associated with increased prevalence of cardiometabolic risk factors, such as type 2 diabetes, dyslipidemia, and hypertension.
- Current recommendations for the prevention of childhood obesity with focus on family-based lifestyle modifications include balanced nutrition, increased physical activity, limited screen time, and healthy sleep patterns.
- Complications and comorbidities of childhood obesity are assessed for with appropriate screening modalities and indications for subspecialty referral.
- The 4-staged treatment model of childhood obesity, which includes prevention plus, structured weight management, comprehensive multidisciplinary intervention, and tertiary care intervention, is reviewed.

INTRODUCTION

Between 2011 and 2014, 17% of US children ages 2 to 19 years met criteria for obesity and 5.8% for extreme obesity.[1] The prevention and treatment of childhood obesity remain public health priorities. Multiple complex factors lead to overweight and obesity in childhood and thereby influence recommendations for management. Although a comprehensive discussion is beyond the scope of this article, it is important to understand the external factors that shape patient behaviors and decision-making.[2,3] The six-Cs is a useful ecological model that recognizes that both environmental and genetic influences contribute to the development of childhood obesity and includes the cell, child, clan, community, country, and culture.[2] The cell represents genetic influences and biological factors that predispose toward

Disclosure Statement: The author has no financial obligations relevant to the article to disclose.
Hasbro Children's Hospital and Rhode Island Hospital, 593 Eddy Street, Providence, RI 02903, USA
E-mail address: kanderson5@lifespan.org

obesity. The child sphere includes personal and behavioral characteristics, such as self-regulation, media exposure, and sleep. The clan refers to the family unit and includes parenting styles, responsive feeding practices, and household routines.[2,3] The community encompasses a broad scope, including peers, schools, childcare, access to healthy food, and safe places to play. Country involves public policies that influence access to healthy nutrition and physical activity, such as in schools and other community institutions. Finally, culture refers to overarching cultural and societal norms concerning nutrition and physical activity.[2,3]

In this ecological context, childhood obesity prevention strategies and family-based multidisciplinary comprehensive behavioral treatment of obesity engage children and their families to make healthy behavioral changes within their control. Clinical collaboration with community programs and resources improves access to healthy foods and safe places to play.[4] Support for public health initiatives and public policies can improve funding for evidence-based prevention strategies while also securing reimbursement for the treatment of childhood obesity.

DIAGNOSIS AND DEFINITIONS OF PEDIATRIC OVERWEIGHT AND OBESITY

Overweight and obesity are defined by using the body mass index (BMI; the weight in kilograms divided by the square of the height in meters) and the Centers for Disease Control and Prevention growth charts for age and sex-specific BMI for children older than 2 years of age. The BMI should be calculated and plotted at least annually during well child visits and/or sick visits.[5] During childhood growth, the range of normal BMI changes with age. An adiposity nadir typically occurs between ages 4 to 6, followed by adiposity rebound and subsequent increase in BMI through adolescence.[6] For this reason, standardized BMI percentiles for age and sex are used, rather than absolute BMI values, to define overweight and obesity in children in contrast to the adult population.

Overweight is classified if the BMI is greater than or equal to 85th percentile but less than 95th percentile for age and sex. Obesity is classified if the BMI is greater than or equal to 95th percentile for age and sex. Definitions vary to some extent with regard to classifying higher degrees of obesity (**Table 1**).[1,5,7]

An Endocrine Society Clinical Practice Guideline published in March 2017 recommends classifying children as obese if the BMI is greater than or equal to 95th percentile for age and sex and as extremely obese if the BMI is greater than or equal to 120% of the 95th percentile for age and sex or greater than or equal to 35 kg/m²; however, it does not further classify extreme obesity.[5] Other groups categorize extreme obesity using class II and class III obesity to resemble adult classifications.[7,8] Recent

Table 1	
Classification of overweight and obesity in childhood	
Overweight	BMI is $\geq$85th percentile but <95th percentile for age and sex
Obesity	
Class I	BMI is $\geq$95th percentile for age and sex
Extreme Obesity	
Class II obesity	BMI is $\geq$120% of the 95th percentile for age and sex or $\geq$35 kg/m², whichever is lower
Class III obesity	BMI is $\geq$140% of the 95th percentile for age and sex or $\geq$40 kg/m², whichever is lower

Data from Refs.[1,5,7]

guidelines recommend against using a BMI greater than or equal to 99th percentile for age and sex to define higher degrees of obesity. Notably, studies have shown an association between higher degrees of obesity in children and an increased prevalence of cardiometabolic risk factors, demonstrating the clinical significance of refining the classification of obesity.[8] Children with class II obesity may be at higher risk for abnormal high-density lipoprotein (HDL) levels, and elevated systolic blood pressure and glucose. Children with class III obesity are at higher risk for elevated triglycerides, diastolic blood pressure, and glycated hemoglobin.[8]

PREVALENCE AND INCIDENCE OF PEDIATRIC OVERWEIGHT AND OBESITY IN THE UNITED STATES

The prevalence of obesity in the United States has increased dramatically over the past 30 years. According to data from the National Health and Nutrition Examination Survey in 2013 through 2014, 17.4% of children ages 2 to 19 years met criteria for class I obesity.[7] Of these children, 6.3% met criteria for class II obesity and 2.4% met criteria for class III obesity. The prevalence was higher in older children across all classes of obesity. For instance, 20.9% of children ages 12 to 19 years met criteria for class I obesity compared with 9.2% of children ages 2 to 5 years. Additionally, 9.5% of children ages 12 to 19 years met criteria for class II obesity and 4.3% met criteria for class III obesity. The categories are not mutually exclusive (ie, children who met criteria for class I obesity include all children with a BMI ≥95th percentile).[7] When comparing obesity data from 1999 through 2014, there has been a significant increase in all classes of obesity for children ages 2 to 19 years.[7] The prevalence of obesity is influenced by race and ethnicity. Data from 2011 through 2014 demonstrate a higher prevalence of obesity in Hispanic (21.9%) and non-Hispanic black (19.5%) children compared with non-Hispanic white (14.7%) children.[1] For adolescents ages 12 to 19 years, non-Hispanic black girls (12.7%) and boys (10.7%), and Hispanic girls (8.3%) and boys (9.2%), had a higher prevalence of extreme obesity compared with non-Hispanic white girls (7.4%) and boys (5.9%).[1]

Incidence data for childhood obesity are more limited but indicate that obesity tracks from a young age. The Early Childhood Longitudinal Study, Kindergarten Class of 1998 to 1999 found that annual incidence of obesity for children ages 5 to 14 years in this cohort was highest at younger ages. Children who entered kindergarten as overweight were 4 times more likely than their normal-weight peers to develop obesity by the eighth grade.[9] These data validate obesity prevention initiatives targeted toward children younger than 9 years of age.[5,9]

PREVENTION OF OBESITY IN CHILDREN AND ADOLESCENTS

Pediatricians regularly provide anticipatory guidance about age-appropriate nutrition and physical activity at routine well child visits, with additional monitoring and intervention when needed. Obesity prevention efforts should focus on healthy family-based lifestyle modifications rather than on weight. As such, child and adolescent psychiatrists, psychologists, and other pediatric mental health providers can play a pivotal role in prevention efforts. When counseling adolescents, providers should promote a positive body image and discourage dieting. Families should be encouraged to talk about healthy eating and ways to stay physically active rather than talking about weight. Parents should be encouraged to be healthy role models for their children.[10]

Current recommendations about target behaviors for the prevention of childhood obesity include[5,10–12]

Beverages
- Avoid sugar-sweetened beverages (ie, soda, ice teas, sports drinks, energy drinks, and juice drinks).
- Limit consumption of 100% fruit juices to appropriate portion sizes.[13]
  - Children less than 12 months of age should not drink juice unless clinically indicated.
  - Children 1 through 3 years of age should limit juice intake to 4 ounces per day.
  - Children 4 through 6 years of age should limit juice intake to 4 to 6 ounces per day.
  - Children 7 through 18 years of age should limit juice intake to 8 ounces per day.
- Encourage children to drink low-fat milk and plain tap water.[14]
  - Children less than 12 months of age should not drink cow's milk.
  - Children 1 through 2 years of age should drink whole milk because fat is needed for healthy growth and development. However, in the context of obesity or strong family history of obesity, dyslipidemia, or other cardiovascular risk factors then reduced fat (2%) milk is recommended.
  - Children older than age 2 years should transition to low-fat (1%) or fat-free milk.

Foods and eating habits
- Incorporate a healthy diet made up of foods with low caloric density (vegetables, fruits, whole grains, low-fat dairy products, lean meats, lean fish, and legumes).
- Limit foods with high caloric density (fat-rich meats, fried foods, baked goods, sweets, cheeses, and oil-based sauces).
- Eat breakfast daily.
- Encourage family meals in which parents and children eat together while sitting at a table without distractions (no television or other electronics).
- Limit eating out at restaurants, particularly fast food restaurants.

Physical activity, screen time, and sleep
- Encourage at least 60 minutes of moderate to vigorous physical activity daily.
- Limit noneducational screen time to less than 2 hours per day.
- Remove televisions and other media from the bedroom.
- Foster healthy sleep patterns.

Motivational interviewing (MI) can be used in both primary care and specialized settings for the prevention and management of childhood obesity. This "is a patient-centered communication style that uses specific techniques such as reflective listening, autonomy support, shared decision-making, and eliciting change talk."[15] The efficacy of MI for the management of childhood overweight or obesity in a primary care setting was assessed in a randomized controlled trial involving 42 practices in the Pediatric Research in Office Settings Network of the American Academy of Pediatrics. MI was delivered by primary care providers to parents of overweight children ages 2 through 8 years with the primary outcome measure of BMI percentile at 2-year follow-up. The practices were randomly assigned to 1 of 3 groups: group 1 was usual care, group 2 involved 4 provider-led MI counseling sessions, and group 3 involved 4 provider-led MI sessions and 6 MI sessions led by a registered dietician. Target behaviors assessed included consumption of snack foods, sweetened beverages, fruits, and vegetables, screen time, and physical activity. At 2-year follow-up, BMI percentile for groups 1, 2, and 3 were 90.3%, 88.1%, and 87.1%, respectively. BMI percentile differences for groups 1, 2, and 3 were 1.8%, 3.8%, and 4.9%, respectively. Results demonstrated that overweight children who were in group 3 (provider-led and registered dietician-led MI sessions) showed a statistically significant reduction in BMI percentile compared with group 1 (usual care) with a net difference between the 2 groups of 3.1% BMI percentile units.[15]

ASSESSMENT FOR COMORBIDITIES

The medical assessment of pediatric obesity includes obtaining a history of parental obesity, as well as a family medical history of possible related health conditions (eg, type 2 diabetes mellitus (DM), hypertension, and dyslipidemia). A careful review of systems and physical examination is important in assessing for obesity-related comorbidities, which affect almost every organ system.[11]

Pulmonary and sleep problems associated with obesity include obstructive sleep apnea, obesity hypoventilation syndrome, and asthma. Children who exhibit daytime somnolence, poor attention, frequent loud snoring, and/or pauses in breathing during the night should alert clinicians to assess for obstructive sleep apnea by ordering polysomnography. Treatment can include tonsillectomy and, if more severe, a pulmonologist can assess the need for continuous positive airway pressure therapy. Left untreated, sequelae of obstructive sleep apnea include right ventricular hypertrophy and pulmonary hypertension.[11]

Cardiometabolic risk factors associated with obesity include elevated systolic and diastolic blood pressure, insulin resistance, type 2 diabetes, and dyslipidemia. An increase in severity of obesity has been associated with a higher risk of certain cardiometabolic risk factors, including low HDL cholesterol levels, high systolic and diastolic blood pressures, high triglyceride levels, and elevated glycated hemoglobin levels.[8]

Blood pressure should be regularly assessed in the office setting using a properly sized blood pressure cuff. Elevated blood pressure levels are defined using tables from the National Heart, Lung, and Blood Institute according to age, gender, and height percentiles. Hypertension in children is diagnosed when 3 or more readings higher than the 95th percentile for either systolic or diastolic are documented.[11] Referral to a pediatric nephrologist or cardiologist is warranted to assess the role for medication.

The Expert Panel on Integrated Guidelines for Cardiovascular Health and Risk Reduction in Children and Adolescents recommends universal lipid screening for children ages 9 to 11 years and for adolescents ages 17 to 21 years.[16] Additionally, a fasting lipid profile should be obtained in children with a BMI greater than or equal to 85th percentile, even in the absence of risk factors. Acceptable, borderline, and elevated cholesterol levels for children and adolescents include[5,11,16]

- Total cholesterol level less than 170 mg/dL is considered acceptable; a level 170 to 199 is borderline high, and a level greater than or equal to 200 mg/dL is high.
- Low-density lipoprotein cholesterol level less than 110 mg/dL is considered acceptable, 110 to 129 is borderline high, and a level greater than or equal to 130 mg/dL is high.
- HDL cholesterol level greater than 45 mg/dL is considered acceptable; a level 40 to 45 mg/dL is borderline low, and a level less than or equal to 40 is considered low.
- Triglyceride levels for children ages of 10 to 19 years of age less than 90 mg/dL is considered acceptable; a level 90 to 129 md/dL is borderline high, and a level greater than or equal to 130 mg/dL is high.

First-line treatment of lipid abnormalities focuses on therapeutic lifestyle changes, including physical activity and reduced-cholesterol diets. If levels remain elevated despite lifestyle changes, referral to a cardiologist or lipid specialist is warranted to assess the role for medication.[11]

Risk factors for type 2 diabetes include a BMI greater than or equal to 85th percentile; a family history of diabetes in first-degree or second-degree relatives; certain races or ethnicities (Native American, African American, Latino, Asian American, and Pacific Islander); signs of insulin resistance, such as acanthosis nigricans; or a condition associated with insulin resistance, such as polycystic ovary syndrome, hypertension, dyslipidemia, or small-for-gestational-age birth weight.[17] Overweight children with 2 or more risk factors should be screened for diabetes every 2 years with a fasting glucose blood test beginning at puberty or 10 years of age.[11] Screening tests for diabetes and prediabetes include a hemoglobin A1C (HbA1C), fasting plasma glucose (no caloric intake for at least 8 hours), and the 2-hour oral glucose tolerance test. Criteria for the diagnosis of diabetes includes an HbA1C level greater than or equal to 6.5%, a fasting plasma glucose greater than or equal to 126 mg/dL, or a 2-hour plasma glucose after a 75-g oral glucose tolerance test greater than or equal to 200 mg/dL. Results should be confirmed by repeat testing unless there are signs of unequivocal hyperglycemia. Criteria for the diagnosis of prediabetes includes a fasting blood glucose of 100 to 125 mg/dL, an HbA1C level of 5.7% to 6.4%, or a 2-hour plasma glucose after a 75-g oral glucose tolerance test of 140 to 199 mg/dL.[17] Although epidemiologic studies to support use of HbA1C levels to diagnose diabetes included only adult populations, the American Diabetes Association continues to recommend its use in children and adolescents.[17] The HbA1C can vary with race or ethnicity, and with medical conditions such as hemoglobinopathies, certain anemias, and conditions with an increased red blood cell turnover.[17] A test result that is diagnostic of diabetes warrants referral to a pediatric endocrinologist. Any testing that is diagnostic of prediabetes is associated with future risk of diabetes.[11]

Other endocrine disorders associated with obesity include polycystic ovary syndrome, hypothyroidism, and primary Cushing syndrome; all warrant evaluation and treatment by a pediatric endocrinologist.[11]

Gastrointestinal problems associated with obesity include nonalcoholic fatty liver disease (NAFLD) and gallstones. Other conditions are worsened by obesity, such as gastroesophageal reflux disease and constipation.[11] NAFLD encompasses a range of liver disease from simple steatosis, to nonalcoholic steatohepatitis, to cirrhosis, to end-stage liver disease.[18] NAFLD has become the most common cause of chronic liver disease in US children and adolescents, with an increased prevalence in the context of the current obesity epidemic.[18] Risk factors for NAFLD include overweight or obesity, consumption of soft drinks (rich in fructose), and waist circumference greater than the 95th percentile for age and sex, as well as family history of obesity, insulin resistance, NAFLD, or type 2 DM.[18] Current recommendations include screening with aspartate aminotransferase (AST) and alanine aminotransferase (ALT) testing every 2 years starting at 10 years of age for children with a BMI greater than or equal to 95th percentile or with a BMI greater than or equal to 85th to 94th percentile with other risk factors.[11] Although the ALT level does not always correlate with histologic abnormalities of NAFLD, it remains a reasonable screening mechanism.[11,18] Abdominal ultrasound is a safe and widely available screening test for fatty liver but cannot consistently differentiate between steatosis and fibrosis.[11,18] The exclusion of other causes of liver disease, as well as liver biopsy, are required for definitive diagnosis of NAFLD.[18] Newer diagnostic tests, such as the FibroScan, are being developed. Diagnostic algorithms exist for the management of children with suspected NAFLD and include recommendations for testing to exclude viral, toxic, metabolic (ie, Wilson disease) and systemic (ie, celiac disease or autoimmune hepatitis) causes of fatty liver.[18] Referral to a pediatric hepatologist or gastroenterologist is warranted for AST or ALT results elevated 2 times normal levels (recent normative values proposed for ALT are $\leq$25 U/L for boys and $\leq$22 U/L for girls).[5,11,18]

A rare neurologic condition for which obesity carries an increased risk is pseudotumor cerebri. Patients present with severe headaches and photophobia with blurred optic disks on funduscopic examination; this requires urgent evaluation by a neurologist.[11] Orthopedic conditions such as Blount disease and slipped capital femoral epiphysis are more common among obese children.[11]

There are numerous psychological complications from obesity in children and adolescents, including poor self-esteem, depression and anxiety, as well as increased risk of eating disorders and substance abuse.[5] Obese youths are more likely to be bullied or teased by peers, and unhealthy family communication patterns about weight also negatively affect self-esteem.[5] In a study investigating the various factors predicting eating-disordered behaviors in early adolescent girls with overweight or obesity, a total of 135 Hispanic and African American girls completed surveys assessing the desire to be thinner, peer weight-related teasing, and disordered eating behaviors, as well as demographics.[19] Results showed that more than half of the study participants had been teased about their weight by girls (52%) and by boys (60%). This study showed a direct association between peer weight-related teasing and weight-control behaviors, binge and purge behaviors, and emotional eating.[19] In a retrospective cohort study of 179 adolescents newly diagnosed with anorexia nervosa or eating disorder not otherwise specified who were seen in a specialty eating disorder clinic, 36.7% were found to have a BMI history higher than the 85th percentile (overweight group). The overweight group had a decrease in BMI of 5.37 kg/m^2 with a mean duration of illness of 19.86 months by time of eating disorder intake. In contrast, the average-weight group had a decrease in BMI of 3.57 kg/m^2 and mean duration of illness of 11.15 months before eating disorder intake.[20] Early detection and treatment improves the chance of recovery from eating disorders; accordingly, adolescents with eating disorders who have a history of overweight may have a poorer prognosis due to delays in identification.[20,21] As such, primary care and mental health providers should not be falsely reassured by a normal or overweight BMI in patients with precipitous or significant weight loss, and should screen these patients for eating disorder behaviors and cognitions. Due to the increased prevalence of psychological comorbidities in obese children, providers should also regularly screen with questions asking about school absences or refusal, teasing by peers, anxiety, depression, self-injurious behaviors, anger outbursts, sexual activity, substance use, eating disordered behaviors, and family attitudes about weight.[5]

Weight gain and adverse cardiometabolic changes associated with the use of second-generation antipsychotics is a growing health concern in psychiatric populations. The binding affinity between antipsychotics and specific receptor subtypes are thought to contribute to weight gain; 5-HT$_{2C}$ (hydroxytryptamine) receptor antagonism may affect appetite suppression and satiety signals via leptin-mediated pathways and H$_1$ (histamine) antagonism produces mild sedation that may be associated with sedentary behavior.[22] Weight gain tends to be most rapid in the first 12 weeks of treatment; younger patients may also be at increased risk of diabetes.[22] When prescribing atypical antipsychotic medications for children, weight, height, and BMI should be measured at baseline and at each clinical visit. Fasting blood work to screen for diabetes and dyslipidemia should be done at baseline, at 3 months, at 6 months, and then twice yearly with more frequent monitoring in the context of significant weight gain.[23] Patients who are prescribed atypical antipsychotic medications should also be counseled about healthy lifestyles, including balanced nutrition and increased physical activity.[23]

STAGES OF TREATMENT OF OBESITY IN CHILDREN AND ADOLESCENTS

A targeted systematic review for the US Preventive Task Force (USPSTF) found that moderate to high intensity comprehensive behavioral interventions were effective for short-term weight loss in obese and overweight children ages 4 to 18 years.[24] These interventions typically incorporate cognitive and behavioral management techniques with patients and their families to encourage weight loss through sustainable changes in diet and physical activity. Moderate intensity was defined as 26 to 75 hours of contact and high intensity as greater than 75 hours of contact over 6 to 12 months.[24] The USPSTF issued a grade B recommendation to screen all children 6 years of age and older for obesity and refer children with obesity to a comprehensive, intensive behavioral intervention to improve weight status.[25] In 2015, consensus recommendations for the treatment of childhood obesity included[25]

- Family-based comprehensive behavioral treatment to promote healthy lifestyle changes, encourage positive parenting techniques, and apply self-regulatory skills.
- Integrated chronic care model that allows for medical monitoring over time, enables an appropriate longitudinal treatment schedule rather than reliance on acute episodes of care, and promotes inclusion of community resources.
- Multidisciplinary care team that should include a pediatrician or primary care provider, behavioral interventionist, subspecialists as indicated, and a care coordinator.

Experts recommend a step or staged approach for the treatment of childhood obesity that is divided into 4 stages (**Table 2**)[11,26]:

- Prevention Plus
- Structured Weight Management
- Comprehensive Multidisciplinary Intervention
- Tertiary Care Intervention.

Table 2
Stages of treatment for childhood obesity

	Stage of Treatment	Setting
Stage 1	Prevention Plus	Primary care office with primary care provider and trained office staff
Stage 2	Structured Weight Management	Primary care office with primary care provider, trained office staff, and dietician
Stage 3	Comprehensive Multidisciplinary Intervention	Multidisciplinary team experienced in childhood obesity including a behavior counselor, registered dietician, exercise specialist, and primary care provider who monitors medical issues. Consider referral to an established pediatric weight management program.
Stage 4	Tertiary Care Intervention	Multidisciplinary team experienced in childhood obesity including a physician, nurse practitioner, registered dietician, behavioral counselor, and exercise specialist. The team should follow standard clinical protocols for evaluation before, during and after the intervention.

Data from Barlow SE, Expert Committee. Expert committee recommendations regarding the prevention, assessment, and treatment of child and adolescent overweight and obesity: summary report. Pediatrics 2007;120(Suppl 4):S164–92; and Spear BA, Barlow SE, Ervin C, et al. Recommendations for treatment of child and adolescent overweight and obesity. Pediatrics 2007;120(Suppl 4):S254–88.

Stage 1: Prevention Plus

Prevention Plus differs from routine obesity prevention counseling (healthy eating habits, increased physical activity, and limited screen time) in that the goal is improvement in BMI and requires more frequent monitoring. During this stage of treatment, the goal is weight maintenance rather than weight loss with an expected decrease in BMI as the child grows.[11,26] Target behavioral changes include[5,11,26]

- Consume greater than or equal to 5 servings of fruits and vegetables every day.
- Limit or eliminate sugar-sweetened beverages.
- Limit noneducational screen time to less than or equal to 2 hours per day. Encourage removal of any television in the child's bedroom and recommend no television viewing for children younger than age 2 years.
- Engage in greater than or equal to 1 hour of physical activity each day.
- Limit meals eaten at restaurants.
- Eat family meals at the table at least 5 to 6 times per week.
- Eat breakfast daily.
- Allow the child to self-regulate his or her meals and avoid overly restrictive feeding behaviors.
- Consider cultural differences when making these recommendations.

Providers can use MI with families to identify a plan to implement behavioral changes. Physicians and trained office staff can deliver this level of treatment in the primary care office. If there has been no improvement in BMI after 3 to 6 months, the child should be advanced to stage 2, Structured Weight Management.[11,26]

Stage 2: Structured Weight Management

Structured Weight Management incorporates the recommendations of Prevention Plus in a more supportive and structured manner to help children achieve target behavioral changes.[11,26] Stage 2 recommendations include[5,11,26]

- Develop a daily balanced eating plan with small amounts of energy-dense foods.
- Outline structured daily meals and planned snacks (breakfast, lunch, dinner, and 1 or 2 scheduled snacks per day).
- Limit noneducational screen time to less than or equal to 1 hour per day.
- Engage in greater than or equal to 1 hour of physical activity each day.
- Monitor targeted behaviors using logs by patient, family, and/or provider.
- Reinforce achievement of targeted behaviors (rather than weight goals).

Monthly follow-up appointments should occur in the primary care office by a team consisting of the primary care provider, office staff trained in MI, and a dietician who can develop an appropriate and balanced eating plan. Additional resources could include a counselor to assist with parenting skills or family conflict resolution, and an exercise therapist to help develop a sustainable plan for increased physical activity. Implementation of group sessions for this level of treatment can also be considered.[5,11,26]

Stage 3: Comprehensive Multidisciplinary Intervention

Comprehensive Multidisciplinary Intervention requires a higher frequency of office visits and an expansion of the specialists involved in treatment to increase the intensity of behavioral changes. The targeted behavioral changes include those of stage 2 with addition of the following[11,26]:

- Develop a structured dietary and physical activity plan that creates a planned negative energy balance.

- Incorporate a structured behavioral modification program with food and activity monitoring.
- Involve parents in behavioral modification techniques for children younger than 12 years of age.
- Train parents to modify the home environment in a healthy direction.
- Evaluate body measurements, dietary intake, and physical activity at baseline and at regular intervals.
- Schedule frequent office visits with a minimum of weekly visits for 8 to 12 weeks and consideration of monthly visits thereafter.
- Consider group office visits.

Treatment at this stage includes a behavioral counselor, registered dietician, exercise specialist, and a primary care provider for medical monitoring. If available, referral to an established pediatric weight management program should be considered. Weight maintenance or gradual weight loss are goals in this treatment stage. Children ages 2 to 5 should not exceed weight loss of more than 1 pound per month. Older obese children and adolescents should not exceed weight loss of more than 2 pounds per week.[26] If more rapid weight loss is observed (>2 lb/week), children should be screened for eating disordered behaviors, such as meal skipping, purging, excessive exercise, and use of diuretics or laxatives.[26]

Stage 4: Tertiary Care Intervention

Referral for Tertiary Care Intervention is appropriate for some severely obese youths who have unsuccessfully attempted weight loss in a comprehensive multidisciplinary intervention and are willing to continue these lifestyle behavioral modifications. They should have the maturity to understand the risks associated with treatments that can include pharmacotherapy and/or bariatric surgery. Treatment at this stage requires a multidisciplinary team experienced in childhood obesity, including a physician, nurse practitioner, registered dietician, behavioral counselor, and exercise specialist. The team should follow standard clinical protocols for evaluation before, during, and after the intervention.[5,11,26]

Pharmacotherapy for the treatment of pediatric obesity includes Orlistat, which inhibits enteric lipase, leading to fat malabsorption.[11] Orlistat is approved by the US Food and Drug Administration (FDA) for obesity treatment of children ages 12 to 16 years of age, and it is associated with a significant BMI reduction in adolescents by 0.7 to 1.7 kg/m^2. However, long-term patient compliance is problematic due to negative gastrointestinal side-effect profile and need for a before-meal dosing schedule.[5] Sibutramine, a serotonin reuptake inhibitor associated with decreased appetite, had been FDA-approved for the treatment of pediatric obesity for adolescents older than or equal to 16 years of age[11,26]; however, it was withdrawn from the United States in 2010 due to concerns regarding cardiovascular safety.[5] There are several medications that have been recently FDA-approved for the treatment of obesity in adults and are considered appropriate for adolescents 16 years of age or older with a BMI greater than or equal to 30 kg/m^2 or a BMI greater than or equal to 27 kg/m^2 with at least 1 weight-related medical condition, such as hypertension or type 2 DM.[5] Pediatric data for these medications are limited; they should only be prescribed by physicians experienced in the use of antiobesity agents. An Endocrine Society Clinical Practice Guideline published in March 2017 postulates that "pharmacotherapeutic agents not yet approved for the treatment of pediatric obesity should be restricted to large, well-controlled clinical studies."[5]

Metformin is an oral antihyperglycemic medication that is considered first-line treatment of type 2 diabetes. The FDA has approved its use in patients older than 10 years of age and approved the extended release preparation in patients older than 17 years of age.[27] Although metformin is not FDA-approved for obesity treatment, it has been used in children and adolescents who are prescribed atypical antipsychotic medications due to its weight-attenuating properties.[5,27] The Improving Metabolic Parameters of Antipsychotic Child Treatment (IMPACT) study is an ongoing multisite, 6 month, randomized open-label clinic trial of overweight or obese youth between the ages of 8 to 19 years with specific psychiatric diagnoses who have experienced weight gain in the context of antipsychotic treatment in the preceding 3 years.[28] Participants are randomized to 1 of 3 arms:

- Change antipsychotic plus healthy lifestyle education
- Add metformin plus healthy lifestyle education
- Healthy lifestyle education with no medication change.

The primary outcome is to compare weight change among the 3 groups. Secondary outcomes include percentage of body fat, insulin resistance, lipid profile, psychiatric symptom stability, and all-cause and specific-cause discontinuation. The IMPACT study aims to compare the risks and benefits of 2 pharmacologic strategies that may mitigate the weight gain and negative metabolic sequelae of antipsychotic medication use in children.[28]

Metformin reduces hepatic gluconeogenesis, decreases intestinal glucose uptake, and increases peripheral insulin sensitivity in muscle.[27] Adverse side effects include development of vitamin B12 deficiency, gastrointestinal side effects, and lactic acidosis. Metformin has been contraindicated in renal impairment, surgery, the use of contrast agents, liver dysfunction, congestive heart failure, alcoholism, metabolic acidosis, dehydration, and hypoxemia.[27]

Bariatric surgery can be considered for adolescents with extreme obesity with BMI greater than or equal to 40 kg/m^2, or BMI of greater than 35 kg/m^2 and a significant comorbidity (eg, type 2 DM, moderate to severe obstructive sleep apnea, or pseudotumor cerebri) who have failed nonsurgical interventions.[5] Patients should meet the following criteria [5,11,26]:

- Physical examination consistent with Tanner 4 or 5 pubertal development
- Height has reached final or near final adult level
- BMI greater than or equal to 40 kg/m^2, or BMI of greater than 35 kg/m^2 and a significant comorbidity (eg, type 2 DM, moderate to severe obstructive sleep apnea, or pseudotumor cerebri)
- Demonstrated greater than or equal to 6 months of compliance with a formal weight management program and ability to adhere to ongoing lifestyle behavioral modifications
- Psychological evaluation to ensure emotional and cognitive maturity of the patient and family, and that the patient does not have an untreated psychiatric illness.

Surgery is not recommended for preadolescents, patients who are pregnant or breast-feeding or who plan to become pregnant in the 2 years following surgery. Surgery should only be performed by an experienced surgeon in a pediatric bariatric surgery center of excellence that follows standardized clinical protocols before, during, and after the intervention.[5,11,26] A multidisciplinary team should include a bariatric surgeon, pediatric obesity specialist, dietician, mental health professional, program coordinator, and social worker. Patients require lifelong monitoring for complications such as dumping syndrome and adherence to nutritional and vitamin supplement guidelines, as well as annual screening for vitamin and mineral deficiencies. Patients are prescribed vitamin and mineral supplements because deficiencies are common due to changes in absorption and gastric acid production.[5,11] Studies have demonstrated an improvement after bariatric surgery in comorbidities associated with obesity, including insulin sensitivity, sleep apnea, nonalcoholic steatohepatitis, and cardiovascular risk factors. Bariatric surgery can be an effective treatment of extremely obese teenagers and has demonstrated positive effects on life-threatening complications of obesity.[5]

DISCUSSION

The prevention and management of childhood obesity remain a public health priority and entail an integrated chronic care approach to affect significant change. "Integrated care has been defined as being coordinated across professionals, facilities, and support systems; continuous over time and between visits; tailored to needs and preferences of patients/families; and based on shared responsibility between patients/families and caregivers for optimizing health."[29] An integrated care model for childhood obesity promotes engagement and empowerment of patients and their families. Trained providers can facilitate behavior changes in diet and physical activity and refer patients to appropriate community programs, such as recreational facilities and afterschool programs. However, clinical interventions cannot readily succeed without adequate community resources, such as access to healthy food or safe places for physical activity.[4] Affecting behavioral changes on a population level requires public policies and public health initiatives to promote more healthy environments, especially among groups with significant health disparities.[4]

The USPSTF recommends that all children older than age 6 years are screened for obesity and, if clinically indicated, are referred for moderate to high intensity comprehensive behavioral interventions. Notably, moderate intensity was defined as 26 to 75 hours of contact and high intensity as greater than 75 hours of contact over 6 to 12 months.[24] A 2015 consensus panel concluded that these interventions should be family-based and comprehensive, using an integrated chronic care model led by a multidisciplinary team.[25]

Childhood obesity and its associated comorbidities affect most systems of the body and, therefore, affect most medical specialties. A shared understanding of current prevention strategies, lifestyle recommendations, screening guidelines for assessment of comorbidities, and stages of treatment of obesity in children and adolescents will allow all health professionals involved in the care of children to create integrated and collaborative care.

REFERENCES

1. Ogden CL, Carroll MD, Lawman HG, et al. Trends in obesity prevalence among children and adolescents in the United States, 1988-1994 through 2013-2014. JAMA 2016;315(21):2292–9.
2. Harrison K, Bost K, McBride B, et al. Towards a developmental conceptualization of contributors to overweight and obesity in childhood: the six-Cs model. Child Dev Perspect 2011;5(1):50–8.
3. Fiese B, Bost K, McBride BA, et al. Childhood obesity prevention from cell to society. Trends Endocrinol Metab 2013;24(8):375–7.
4. Dietz W, Solomon L, Pronk N, et al. An integrated framework for the prevention and treatment of obesity and its related chronic diseases. Health Aff (Millwood) 2015;34(9):1456–63.

5. Styne D, Arslanian S, Connor EL, et al. Pediatric obesity- assessment, treatment, and prevention: an endocrine society clinical practice guideline. J Clin Endocrinol Metab 2017;102(3):709–57.

6. Lo JC, Maring B, Chandra M, et al. Prevalence of obesity and extreme obesity in children aged 3-5 years. Pediatr Obes 2013;9(3):167–75.

7. Skinner A, Perrin E, Skelton J. Prevalence of obesity and severe obesity in US children, 1999-2014. Obesity 2016;24(3):1116–23.

8. Skinner A, Perrin E, Moss LA, et al. Cardiometabolic risks and severity of obesity in children and young adults. N Engl J Med 2015;373(14):1307–17.

9. Cunningham S, Kramer M, Narayan KM. Incidence of childhood obesity in the United States. N Engl J Med 2014;370(5):403–11.

10. Golden N, Schneider M, Wood C, Committee on Nutrition, Committee on Adolescence, Section on Obesity. Preventing obesity and eating disorders in adolescents. Pediatrics 2016;138(3):e1–10.

11. Barlow S. Expert committee recommendations regarding the prevention, assessment, and treatment of child and adolescent overweight and obesity: summary report. Pediatrics 2007;120:S164–92.

12. Daniels S, Hassink S, Committee of Nutrition. The role of the pediatrician in primary prevention of obesity. Pediatrics 2015;136(1):e275–92.

13. Heyman M, Abrams S, Section on Gastroenterology, Hepatology, and Nutrition, Committee on Nutrition. Fruit juice in infants, children, and adolescents: current recommendations. Pediatrics 2017;139:1–8, e2017–0967.

14. Holt K, Wooldridge N, Story M, et al. Nutrition supervision. In: Bright futures nutrition. 3rd edition. Elk Groove Village (IL): The American Academy of Pediatrics; 2011. p. 17–111.

15. Resnicow K, McMaster F, Bocian A, et al. Motivational interviewing and dietary counseling for obesity in primary care: an RCT. Pediatrics 2015;135(4):649–57.

16. Expert Panel on Integrated Guidelines for Cardiovascular Health and Risk Reduction in Children and Adolescents. Expert panel on integrated guidelines for cardiovascular health and risk reduction in children and adolescents: summary report. Pediatrics 2011;128(Suppl 5):S213–56.

17. American Diabetes Association. Classification and diagnosis of diabetes. Diabetes Care 2016;39(Suppl 1):S13–22.

18. Vajro P, Lenta S, Socha P, et al. Diagnosis of nonalcoholic fatty liver disease in children and adolescents: position pater of the ESPGHAN hepatology committee. J Pediatr Gastroenterol Nutr 2012;54(5):700–13.

19. Olvera N, McCarley K, Matthews-Ewald M, et al. Pathways for disordered eating behaviors in minority girls: the role of adiposity, peer weight-related teasing, and desire to be thinner. The J Early Adolescence 2017;37(3):367–86.

20. Lebow J, Sim L, Kransdorf L. Prevalence of a history of overweight and obesity in adolescents with restrictive eating disorders. J Adolesc Health 2015;56:19–24.

21. van Son G, van Hoeken D, van Furth EF, et al. Course and outcome of eating disorders in a primary care-based cohort. Int J Eat Disord 2010;43(2):130–8.

22. Newall H, Myles N, Ward PB, et al. Efficacy of metformin for prevention of weight gain in psychiatric populations: a review. Int Clin Psychopharmacol 2012;27(2):69–75.

23. Maayan L, Correll C. Weight gain and metabolic risks associated with antipsychotic medications in children and adolescents. J Child Adolesc Psychopharmacol 2011;21(6):517–35.

24. Whitlock E, O'Connor E, Williams SB, et al. Effectiveness of weight management interventions in children: a targeted systematic review for the USPSTF. Pediatrics 2010;125(2):e396–408.
25. Wilfley D, Staiano A, Altman M, et al. Improving access and systems of care for evidence-based childhood obesity treatment: conference key findings and next steps. Obesity 2017;25(1):16–29.
26. Spear B, Barlow S, Ervin C, et al. Recommendations for treatment of child and adolescent overweight and obesity. Pediatrics 2007;120:S254–88.
27. Thomas I, Gregg B. Metformin; a review of its history and future: from lilac to longevity. Pediatr Diabetes 2017;18(1):10–6.
28. Reeves G, Keeton C. Improving metabolic parameters of antipsychotic child treatment (IMPACT) study: rationale, design, and methods. Child Adolesc Psychiatry Ment Health 2013;7:31.
29. Ebbeling C, Antonelli R. Primary care interventions for pediatric obesity: need for an integrated approach. Pediatrics 2015;135(4):757–8.

Domestic Minor Sex Trafficking

Amy Goldberg, MD[a],*, Jessica Moore, BA[b]

KEYWORDS

- Domestic minor sex trafficking (DMST)
- Commercial sexual exploitation of minors (CSEC) • Sexual abuse
- Sexual exploitation • Sexually transmitted infection (STI)

KEY POINTS

- Commercial sexual exploitation of children and child sex trafficking is a major public health issue and a manifestation of the child sexual abuse occurring globally. Recently, these crimes have become increasingly recognized within the United States, where it is known as domestic minor sex trafficking.
- Sexually exploited minors are commonly identified as having psychosocial risk factors, such as histories of abuse or neglect, running away, substance use or abuse, and involvement with child protective services. Youth also suffer a variety of physical and mental health consequences, including posttraumatic stress disorder, depression, anxiety, and suicidality.
- Child psychiatrists and other medical providers have the opportunity to identify, interact, and intervene on behalf of involved and at-risk youth.

DEFINITIONS

Commercial Sexual Exploitation of Children

Commercial sexual exploitation of children (CSEC), also referred to as child sex trafficking or commercial sexual exploitation of youth, is defined as the engagement of minors (<18 years of age) in sexual acts for money, food, shelter, or another valued entity.[1] Sexual acts are broadly defined to include street-based and Internet-based sex, escorting, survival sex, stripping, pornography, or other acts in any venue. The federal Trafficking Victims Protection Act of 2000 states that the identification of minors as victims does not require evidence of threat, force, fraud, or coercion.[1]

CSEC is a broad term that encompasses international, domestic, and transnational sex trafficking. Exploited adolescents can be trafficked across national borders, within a country, a state, or a single neighborhood.[2,3] Using the terminology of CSEC as

Disclosure Statement: The authors have no commercial or financial conflicts of interest or funding sources.

[a] Department of Pediatrics, The Warren Alpert Medical School of Providence, RI 02906, USA;
[b] Hasbro Children's Hospital, Providence, RI 02906, USA
* Corresponding author. 593 Eddy Street, Providence, RI 02903.
E-mail address: agoldberg@lifespan.org

opposed to prostitution reflects a notable shift in the nomenclature and perception of trafficked youth, in which destigmatizing language identifies involved minors as victims instead of criminals.[2,3] Greater awareness of this issue will facilitate a continued appropriate shift away from the disparaging paradigm that portrayed youth as blameworthy criminals and prostitutes, into a conception of these minors as survivors of child sexual abuse.[3]

Domestic Minor Sex Trafficking

There has been increased recognition of a subset of CSEC that identifies a population of victims who are US citizens or lawful permanent residents under the age of 18 years trafficked within United States borders; this is known as domestic minor sex trafficking (DMST).[3,4] The recognition of DMST as a subset of CSEC is important because research has found that risk factors, consequences of involvement, and trafficking experiences differ between domestic and international victims. Muftic and Finn[5] found that, compared with international sex trafficking survivors, domestic sex trafficking survivors had poorer health outcomes (physical injuries, sexually transmitted infections [STIs], mental health issues), histories of child physical and/or sexual abuse, alcohol or drug addiction, and reported suicidal ideations.[5] The information presented in this article focuses on issues related specifically to DMST.

Epidemiology

There are currently no reliable national statistics on the incidence and prevalence of DMST due to the exceptional challenges associated with victim identification.[2] Obtaining accurate data is difficult due to the clandestine nature of these crimes, survivors denying involvement, lack of collaboration across multiple disciplines, and the application of different definitions and laws.[4] The incidence of DMST is believed to be underreported, similar to cases of child sexual abuse.[6] Particularly, there is a paucity of reporting by male victims and by gay, bisexual, transgender, and queer involved youth, due to a hesitancy of disclosures and because most outreach programs focus on female victims.[2,6,7]

It is conservatively estimated that 200,000 US minors are exploited annually with instances reported in all 50 states and the District of Columbia.[8] Furthermore, it is most widely cited that approximately 244,000 to 325,000 children are at risk for sex trafficking each year.[9] The average age a child is recruited is 12 to 14-years-old.[4] A uniform approach to this problem across the country is necessary to fully understand the causes of these crimes, including consistent terminology use, a centralized database, and more frequent and broader screening, particularly in high-risk populations.[2-4]

RISK

Risk factors for involvement in DMST include variables related to involved and at-risk individuals, their relationships with others, the community in which the individual resides, and society at large.[7] The socioecological model is useful in considering the broad range of factors that place people at risk and illustrates how these factors interact within and across levels to increase risk or protection.[10] This model has been adapted to demonstrate the complex forces that may contribute to initial and continued involvement in DMST (**Fig. 1**).[7]

Normative Adolescent Psychosocial Development

By virtue of their normal maturation and developmental stages, adolescents may be at risk of being recruited into DMST involvement.[4] Normal adolescent development

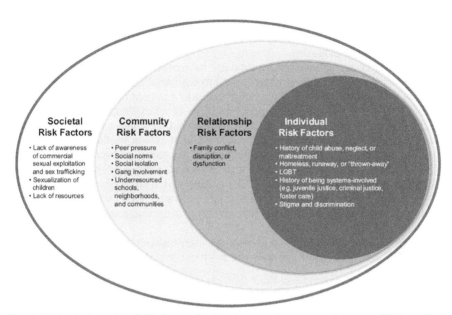

Fig. 1. Ecological model of risk factors for involvement in commercial sex trafficking of minors. LGBT, lesbian, gay, bisexual, and transgender. (*From* Clayton EW, Krugman RD, Simon P. Confronting Commercial Sexual Exploitation and Sex Trafficking of Minors in the United States. Institute of Medicine and National Research Council. Washington, DC: The National Academies Press; 2013; with permission.)

involves the formation of peer relationships, independence from parents, sexual experimentation, impulsivity, risk-taking behaviors, and a sense of invulnerability.[11] Furthermore, youth may be more susceptible to exploitation by traffickers in comparison with adults due to their limited life experience and capacity to consider consequences, lack of psychosocial maturity, and fewer coping mechanisms.[4,7] Detecting exploitative motives and identifying manipulation may be more difficult for adolescents than for adults.[11] Traffickers prey on these normal adolescent vulnerabilities, thereby placing all youth at risk for DMST recruitment and subsequent involvement.[2]

Risk Factors

Although all adolescents are at risk of involvement in sex trafficking, some children are at heightened susceptibility.[4,7,8] Using the ecological model framework, the literature has documented the multiple potential direct and indirect pathways that may trigger initiation into commercial sexual exploitation (see **Fig. 1**).

Individual-Level Factors

The Institute of Medicine and National Research Council list several factors that increase vulnerability at the individual level, including forms of previous maltreatment, disruptions in normative development, involvement of child welfare systems (eg, living in foster care and/or group home), the experience of running away or being homeless, substance use or abuse, psychogenic factors and impaired cognitive function, and the experience of other early adversity.[7] Children with a history of maltreatment, including sexual abuse, physical abuse, and neglect, are at especially high risk of exploitation.[2,4,6] Recent research by Goldberg and colleagues[12] found that patients referred to medical providers for DMST involvement had histories of child maltreatment (90%), consistent with studies that documented 91% to 95% of female victims reported abuse before their exploitation.

Previous sexual abuse histories, in particular, have been identified by youth as a major influencing factor on their sex trafficking involvement.[13,14] There are several reasons that may explain the correlation between prior maltreatment and initiation into DMST. Stoltz and colleagues[13] suggest that some children who are sexually victimized develop psychologically and emotionally in ways that create a propensity toward later engagement in high-risk sexual behaviors, such as sex trafficking. In support, Steel and Herlitz[14] argue that child sexual abuse is a possible indirect pathway to sexual risk behavior, with psychological symptoms such as depression, poor self-esteem, and posttraumatic stress disorder (PTSD) leading to future risk behavior. Negative consequences may result from an abuse history such as emotional avoidance behaviors (eg, self-harm, substance abuse, running away), in turn increasing an adolescent's susceptibility to sexual exploitation.[7,14]

The following quote is taken directly from an interview with a patient seen in follow-up for DMST who was asked whether she still thought about engaging in trafficking:

I still think about it. I didn't feel like it [trafficking] was any different than my life. It was something that always happened, the only difference was that I was benefiting financially.

The experiences of running away, being homeless, and living in foster care or congregate care environments are also a risk factor for involvement in DMST.[7,15,16] Survivors cited chronic homelessness or lack of stable housing as a particularly significant factor in their susceptibility to the recruitment efforts of their traffickers.[15–17] Reasons that link homelessness to sex trafficking involvement range from a lack of resources for basic needs (eg, food, shelter) to the need for social connection and stability.[16,17] Often, adolescents who run away or are systems-involved come from environments with impaired parental supervision, poverty, neglect, and abuse.[2,9] Further, these adolescents may live in settings where they are at greater risk of victimization because they are more accessible to potential traffickers or peers involved in trafficking (eg, congregate care).

Studies have also indicated that substance abuse is intrinsically linked to runaway behavior, child maltreatment, and exchanging sex for money, specifically survival sex.[17,18] Adolescents who experience abuse and/or neglect may use drugs to cope with negative experiences at home or to relieve symptoms of depression or anxiety. Moore and colleagues[19] found that during history taking and/or at their medical visit, most patients (92%) reported alcohol and substance use or abuse when a disclosure of DMST was made. Preexisting substance use may be a risk factor for youth involvement due to decreased inhibitions and impaired judgment, or it may be used as a recruitment tactic by traffickers promising to supply the youth's addiction.[20]

Relationship-Level Factors

A minor's close relationships, including their family and peers, may increase the risk of engagement in DMST. This may occur directly, such as cases in which involvement in DMST is introduced and endorsed by parents, siblings, peers, and/or significant others.[7] Relationship factors may also occur indirectly; minors who come from dysfunctional families (parental substance abuse, domestic violence) are susceptible to DMST because their living environments often involve impaired parental supervision and support, neglect, and abuse.[5,7] Goldberg and colleagues[12] found that most of their cohort of youth who were involved or suspected to be involved lived at home (68%), and 30% experienced domestic violence and 59% had parents who abused substances. Youth who experience family conflict and/or have unstable housing are more likely to run away, use or abuse substances, and engage in other high-risk behaviors, thereby increasing their likelihood to engage in survival sex[16,17] and be at elevated risk of commercial sexual exploitation.[2,4,6]

Child maltreatment and family dysfunction may result in a youth's disrupted development, defined as life events that disturb normative adolescent development or expose youth to adult responsibilities prematurely.[7] Wickrama and Diana[21] describe the rush-to-adulthood perspective that links precocious transitions to early sexual activity; teenage pregnancy; and negative long-term emotional, behavioral, and physical health outcomes. Additionally, impaired attachment and reactive attachment disorder, in particular, are frequently seen in children who have inconsistent, abusive, or neglectful care in their early childhood. The child develops disorganized attachment patterns and subsequent inability to form secure and potentially healthy relationships.[22] Given the high rates of prior maltreatment associated with this vulnerable adolescent population, it is not surprising that many youth run away from home and feel the need to form relationships regardless of their appropriateness or safety.

Community-Level Factors

Communities can shape perceptions about the types of opportunities available for social mobility, ideas about legitimate means of employment, and beliefs about the acceptability of sexual behaviors; these norms can influence the behaviors of traffickers and victims.[7] Cobbina and Oselin[23] found that 40% of interviewed female sex workers described sex trafficking as normal in their neighborhood and a means of obtaining income. Other community-level factors include the existence of adult sex workers and sex trafficked minors already working near the area, the presence of exploiters or sex establishments (eg, saunas and massage parlors), and a greater population of sex-buyers. Moreover, environments with high rates of crime, police corruption, adult prostitution, and transient men (eg, truckers, members of the military) seem to have an increased risk of sexual exploitation.[2,7,22]

Poverty is another well-documented community risk factor for involvement in DMST.[4,7] Living in poverty and disadvantaged conditions has been linked to high-risk sexual behaviors and earlier onset of sexual activity.[7,24] Although there is a need for quantitative evidence linking poverty to involvement in DMST, qualitative reports from law enforcement, social service providers, and others working in the anti-trafficking movements have corroborated this correlation.[7,25]

Societal-Level Factors

Societal norms and expectations about sexual behaviors, including sexual consent and coercion, plus standards regarding minors, gender, sexual orientation, and race or ethnicity, also contribute to the risk for DMST involvement.[7] Societal risk factors may include glorification of pimp culture, objectification of women and girls, and gender bias.[2] These factors shape the expectations of youth, potential traffickers, and sex buyers in regard to how girls and women should be treated within their society.[26] Furthermore, the sexualization of children, particularly girls, may play a role in the risk for DMST by normalizing sex trafficking of minors and sex-buyer demand for younger children. The use of the Internet and social media enables the mass production of these norms that are infiltrated into society.[5,8]

RECRUITMENT

The psychosocial context and aforementioned risk factors place youth at increased susceptibility to the tactics used by traffickers to recruit youth for commercial sexual exploitation. Prior research suggests that traffickers often use recruiters to identify and target youth by frequenting their hang out locations and befriending potential victims.[2,4] Traffickers often use a myriad of coercive techniques to persuade and manipulate youth to become involved: promises of money and items, enticing lifestyles and careers (eg, modeling), feeling empowered, and having a sense of belonging.[2,19] Exploiters may also use physical force, legal threats, or show intimacy and affection toward victims. In a case review of 79 female youth, Reid[27] found that the most common entrapment schemes included flattery and romance, becoming an ally and building trust, normalizing sex, isolating youth, and preying on intellectually disabled minors.

Traffickers may have a relationship to the victim, such as being a family member, a friend, or peer, or may present themselves as empathetic romantic partners, whereas others may be a stranger to the victim.[4,19] Regardless of the relationship and tactics used, a complex dynamic is created between exploiters and their victims through manipulating a youth's specific vulnerabilities and needs.

Peer Networks

Despite the widespread belief that adults are directly responsible for the entry of youth into sexual exploitation, research on recruitment through peer networks shows that this experience is more common than often realized.[28,29] Curtis and colleagues[29] revealed that 44% to 68% of youth in the sample reported initiation by their perceived friends. Moore and colleagues[19] found that victims commonly reported their trafficker to be a friend (28%). Individuals whom victims consider friends may work as surrogate recruiters for traffickers by modeling this behavior and normalizing participation in sex trafficking. Many peers are appointed by the trafficker to the role of what is termed a bottom.[30,31] A bottom is a woman or girl who befriends other girls, recruits or trains them, and provides discipline (ie, violence).[19,30]

Peer-to-peer recruitment methods may also be reinforced by peer pressure and society's glamorization of the sex industry.[7,29] The barrage of media sources and popular music depict a conception of pimps and so-called hos and feature sexualized images of girls or women, which normalize sexualization and engagement in sex trafficking.[2,9,29]

Social Media

Social media plays an integral role in the complex dynamics of adolescent recruitment and the solicitation of sex-buyers or clients.[29,32,33] Exploiters use online and digital technologies for recruiting, grooming, and advertising victims for the purposes of DMST.[33] Social media is often the means through which recruiters prey on vulnerable youth by establishing a friendship or romantic relationship, as well as in connecting victims with each other. This makes exiting from DMST an even greater challenge because survivors may remain connected online.[29,33]

Grooming

Traffickers often target vulnerable adolescents using a variety of sophisticated coercive techniques.[2,3,22] In child sexual abuse, the process by which a child molester overcomes a child's resistance to sex and elicits cooperation in a progressive manner is referred to as grooming. In building this relationship, the molester may offer love and/or items with the ultimate goal of gaining the child's trust.[30,34] Moreover, the act of grooming develops a relationship bonding perpetrators and youth, and is used in the recruitment process for DMST. Exploiters may glamorize and normalize sexual acts through the use of jokes and luring them via bottoms. Isolation, abduction, and coercion via drugs and by debt bondage are other grooming techniques.[7] Commonly, the trafficker will establish a relationship with the adolescent similar to a romantic partner or friend.[29] Subsequent techniques, such as fear and coercion, are used to keep the involved youth from leaving.

This 15-year-old female patient's personal account, during her initial evaluation for DMST, is a clinical example of how a relationship may be developed with a trafficker:

> I was walking home from school and he pulled up to me in his car and asked me if anyone ever told me I should model. He asked me for my phone number and then he texted me every day, like 50 times a day, little things like "how's your day going?" and "how's school?" After about 2 months, we started dating and then he would pick me up and we would go to a motel and have sex during school-...The first time he had me go to a hotel with another girl, she was working not me and he beat her up in front of me because she didn't want to do certain things. I knew I would have to do it soon too.

ENMESHMENT
Intimate Partner Violence

The relationship that develops between the minor and exploiter in DMST is not dissimilar to that seen in cases of intimate partner violence (IPV).[3] In fact, the Power and Control Wheel developed by Pence and Paymar[35] for IPV is often used to demonstrate the dynamics of establishing and maintaining relationships between victims of DMST and their traffickers. Entrapment and enmeshment tactics used by sex traffickers share several commonalities with those of batterers, such as controlling victims through violence, shame, and intimidation.[2] These tactics eventually undermine the adolescent's ability to act autonomously, keeping involved youth under the control of their exploiters.[2,7]

Trauma Bonding

The colluding effects of disrupted childhood development by experiences of maltreatment, in conjunction with the calculated exploitative methods of sex traffickers, facilitate the creation of trauma bonding between the victim and his or her trafficker.[36] Trauma bonds are a dynamic, cyclical state in which victims form a powerful emotional attachment to their abusive partners.[3,35] Dutton and Painter[37] identified 2 conditions that are necessary for victim and abuser trauma bonding to occur: (1) a severe power imbalance causing the victim to feel increasingly helpless and vulnerable and (2) intermittent abuse that alternates with positive or neutral interactions. Grooming techniques (eg, flattery, building trust, normalizing sex) are used to establish the perception that victims are in a consensual and special relationship with their trafficker; thus they develop feelings of loyalty, making some youth not perceive their victimization.[2,4,7] The relationship descends into intimidation and violence, in which enmeshment techniques include blackmailing, shaming, financial control, and isolation. As a result, the youth is willing to do what the exploiter asks, including engagement in DMST, to preserve the relationship.

Retrafficking

There are challenges faced by adolescents trying to escape their exploitation, including financial difficulties, drug dependency, barriers to finding employment, abusive or dysfunctional home environments, placement in group homes or foster care, criminal convictions, and manipulative exploiters. Traffickers may continue to use past recruitment techniques (eg, substance use, intimacy, violence) on victims to regain control in the face of an adolescent trying to exit their involvement in DMST.[7] Youth may also return to the same circumstances that made them vulnerable initially (eg, lack of stable home, abuse), perpetuating an increased likelihood of retrafficking. It is possible that the longer minors are engaged in DMST, the more the patterns of behavior that contributed to their vulnerability become intractable, thus making it more difficult for them to exit. This phenomenon is particularly evident among women and girls who have lost contact with family and friends, whose most direct peer groups also are also involved in DMST, or who may have an ongoing drug dependency.[7]

CONSEQUENCES OF INVOLVEMENT

Sex trafficking is a particularly brutal and dehumanizing crime involving a range of abuses and traumas, resulting in multiple acute and chronic physical and psychological consequences. Approximately 95% of trafficked women and adolescents have reported physical and/or sexual violence.[2,4,12,29] Adverse physical outcomes include injuries from violence (bruises, concussions, fractures, lacerations), infections (STIs, including human immunodeficiency virus and pelvic inflammatory disease), gynecologic issues (repeat unintended pregnancies or abortions, vaginal lacerations, and hemorrhaging), untreated chronic conditions, malnourishment, and poor dental care.[2,38]

Less research is available on the mental health sequelae of this abuse. However, given the psychologically abusive nature of DMST involvement, many victims report PTSD, other anxiety disorders, depression, suicidal ideation, psychosomatic illness, trauma bonding, drug or alcohol addictions, and eating disorders.[7] Goldberg and colleagues[12] found that most patients (66%) had a previously documented psychiatric diagnosis and 46% required a psychiatric admission in the year before referral for DMST. More than half of patients (54%) described previous and current self-injurious behaviors, 59% of patients reported previous suicidal ideation, and 20% reported current suicidal ideation.[12] Importantly, when interpreting these high rates, psychiatric impairment may be a consequence of DMST involvement, and may also function indirectly in a youth's risk and subsequent engagement in sex trafficking (Fig. 2).

A consequence of DMST involvement may also be substance abuse; youth may be forced to use illicit drugs by traffickers as a means of coercion and control. Youth may use alcohol and/or drugs as a coping mechanism to dull the trauma experienced during the period of exploitation.[17] Similar to other psychiatric illnesses, substance use or abuse may function as both a risk factor for and consequence of involvement in DMST (see Fig. 2).

BARRIERS TO CARE

Patients seek medical attention but are often not identified because they infrequently self-disclose involvement to providers and do not consistently present with evidence of involvement (eg, found trafficking by law enforcement).[2,38] Therefore, at-risk or victimized patients are treated solely for their immediate health issues (eg, drug or alcohol abuse, STIs, suicidal ideation, running away from congregate care settings), only to be placed at continued risk or perpetration for DMST victimization.[2,38] Youth who are not recognized within a medical setting represent missed opportunities for identification and intervention.

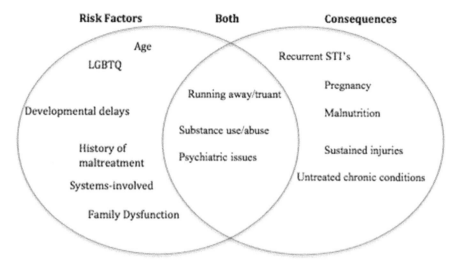

Risk Factors   **Both**   **Consequences**

Age

LGBTQ

Recurrent STI's

Running away/truant

Pregnancy

Developmental delays

Malnutrition

Substance use/abuse

History of
maltreatment

Psychiatric issues

Sustained injuries

Systems-involved

Untreated chronic conditions

Family Dysfunction

Fig. 2. Risk factors and consequences of involvement in DMST.

Given the complex psychological factors involved in DMST, obtaining an accurate history and assessment of trafficked youth may be difficult. Sexually exploited minors may distrust the clinician, may have a desire to protect the perpetrator, and may fear retribution from their exploiter.[4] Many victims have an overwhelming distrust of authority figures based on histories of child maltreatment, abandonment by caregivers, and prior involvement with child protective services and/or law enforcement.[4,5] Moreover, exploited youth may not realize they are being victimized and can be hesitant or unable to describe their traumatic experiences. Shame and stigma have been described as major barriers to victims seeking mental health services.[4,7] Therefore, providers should interview the youth alone, keeping in mind that they may be accompanied to health visits by an exploiter. Due to these aforementioned reasons, DMST patients may not be inclined, especially initially, to communicate openly about their involvement.

In conjunction with barriers that make victim identification difficult, survey studies have found that providers are ill-equipped to identify and manage sex trafficked patients due to limited knowledge of, confidence in, training with, and awareness of DMST.[39–41] Rhode Island pediatricians (86%) described having received 0 hours of training on DMST.[39] Beck and colleagues[40] found that 67% of providers with no training were more likely to have lower levels of knowledge on sex trafficking and noted less confidence in their ability to identify victims. In addition to medical providers, multiple systems (eg, child protection agencies, law enforcement) may be involved in the response to victims of commercial sexual exploitation and sex trafficking of minors. Thus, all professionals who work with victims, including physical health and mental health providers, need standardized training and education on how to appropriately identify and respond to the issue of DMST.

IDENTIFICATION
Signs of Involvement in Domestic Minor Sex Trafficking

To improve the identification of DMST victims, providers should be aware of potential physical, psychological, and medical indicators commonly associated with these

Table 1
Potential indicators of involvement in domestic minor sex trafficking

Social-Environmental Signs	Psychological Signs	Physical Signs
History of running away from home	Appears withdrawn, depressed, fearful	Evidence of physical abuse
History of child protective services	Youth is guarded and does not trust authority figures	Tattoos that indicate branding
Unexplained or multiple absences from home, school, or group home (may be hours to weeks)	Substance use or abuse: drugs and alcohol	Multiple and/or recurrent STIs, pelvic inflammatory disease, multiple sexual partners
Has expensive items or large amounts of money	Person accompanying youth appears controlling or forceful	History of pregnancy and/or abortion
	Provides inconsistent or vague demographic information	Malnutrition, wound infections, other infections
	Legal insecurity: forced illegal activities	Dressed in inappropriate clothing
	Suicidal ideation	Self-harm injuries

victims. For example, screening for DMST should include inquiring about the origin of tattoos incidentally noted during physical examination or visible during any clinical interaction (**Table 1**).

Screening Questions

When a clinician decides to screen a patient for DMST, it is recommended that questions are prefaced with establishing a bridge of understanding between provider and patient. For example, a useful technique involves leading with, "I have patients who are involved in selling or trading sex for things like (blank)." This blank can then be filled in with commodities that the evaluator deems potentially relevant to the child based on the evaluation (eg, a place to stay if evaluating a child who has run away, drugs for a patient who is known to use substances, or money). After the clinician states these examples, the patient is asked if he or she knows about any such exchanges involving sex and something of value (ie, sex trafficking). If the child acknowledges knowing about trafficking, the evaluator might then ask a follow-up question more proximal to the patient, such as whether the patient knows an acquaintance or a friend who has engaged in this activity, "Have any of your friends been asked to have sex in exchange for something they wanted or needed?" If again the patient answers affirmatively, then the clinician can move on to asking more specific questions regarding the patient's involvement. Beginning with a general discussion about sex trafficking and asking increasingly proximal questions in this manner is often referred to as a funnel method. This can be particularly effective in overcoming discomfort, shame, and guilt for the potential victim, thereby more effectively facilitating disclosure. Furthermore, the clinician can gauge the amount of knowledge the patient has about DMST and establish their level of risk. Engaging in a conversation with the youth pertaining to specific issues relevant to the patient and avoiding a list of screening questions is also recommended. Currently, a uniform screening tool does not exist; however, the following questions have been adapted from Greenbaum and Crawford-Jakubiak[2]:

1. Has anyone ever asked you to have sex with another person?
2. Has anyone ever asked you to have sex in exchange for something you wanted or needed (money, food, shelter, or other items)?

3. Has anyone ever taken sexual pictures of you or posted such pictures on the Internet?

Importantly, that if the patient acknowledges knowing about sex trafficking and/or knowing someone who has been involved, but denies personal involvement, there is still an opportunity to provide preventive education about the dangers of involvement. Additionally, this clinical interaction establishes for the adolescent that the clinician can provide a safe clinical space to discuss the topic in the future.

INTERVENTIONS

Given the prevalence of psychosocial issues, trauma, and other mental health disorders associated with this vulnerable adolescent population, child psychiatrists and other mental health providers are uniquely positioned to identify involved and at-risk youth, and engage in prevention, treatment, and advocacy. Studies conducted with both domestic and foreign survivors of sex trafficking suggest that health care providers saw 28% to 88% of survivors at least once during the time they were trafficked.[12,38] Goldberg and colleagues[12] found that more than one-fourth (28%) of the presenting concerns during previous medical visits were related to psychiatric issues, including suicide attempts, bolstering the association between DMST and mental health problems. Health care providers, including child psychiatrists, have the opportunity to intervene and manage patients at-risk for or involved in DMST.

Trauma-Focused Cognitive Behavioral Therapy

Recent literature has cited trauma-informed services (eg, cognitive therapy, exposure therapy) as a potentially effective treatment option for many patients involved in CSEC; however, no prospective case control studies currently exist.[25,42] Cohen and colleagues[43] described trauma-focused cognitive behavioral therapy (TF-CBT) as a therapy modality to address complex trauma experienced by sex trafficked minors, by identifying commonalities among commercially sexually exploited youth and youth with complex trauma. Commonalities include experiencing multiple interpersonal trauma experiences, high levels of PTSD symptoms, elevated levels of externalizing behavior problems, affective dysregulation, negative self-concept, and interpersonal dysfunction. Health care providers should emphasize a safe and supportive environment while integrating caregiver involvement and behavioral strategies to reduce risk-taking behavior.[43] A limitation to this intervention is that TF-CBT requires that a caregiver is successfully integrated into the therapy, which many victims of DMST do not have. Therefore, identifying a trusted and supportive adult for these youth to engage with in this treatment modality should be an alternate strategy.

Education

Teaching youth, particularly high-risk adolescents, how to distinguish between healthy and unhealthy relationships may provide them with the skills to recognize and withstand the manipulation of sex traffickers. Numerous agencies with empirically informed psychoeducational programs exist around the United States with curricula to teach girls how to recognize and avoid the recruitment tactics of exploiters and, more generally, about potentially harmful relationships and self-empowerment. As previously identified, provider's lack of knowledge and training is a barrier to care for these youth. Therefore, several of these agencies also offer workshops and curricula aimed at training professionals about victim identification and improving provider response to exploited youth.[44]

Establishing a Medical Home

The serious consequences associated with sex trafficking demonstrate the importance of health care providers providing a consistent medical home. Compared with a dedicated mental health setting, a medical home where the youth's physical complaints are addressed may be less associated with potential stigma of mental health treatment. It may be an easier way to begin interventions with involved youth, and teens may perceive interactions in medical contexts as being less confrontational than those mental health contexts. For example, providing a full physical examination and communicating with the patient about the physical findings can begin to address the patient's concern that his or her body is damaged or abnormal after repeated physical and sexual trauma. With further discussion over the course of multiple visits, medical providers should establish that they can be a trusted, nonjudgmental, and professional, with the patient's health and safety as their priority. With this established trust, referral to mental health providers can effectively occur. A preexisting collaboration and shared interest in treating these complicated youth between mental health and medical providers, ideally where professionals are colocated or able to easily share information, best serves these patients. Involved youth benefit from consistency in messaging, concretely associating the medical and psychological consequences of DMST, and unified recommendations.

Multidisciplinary Approach

To effectively treat the complex and multifaceted needs of these vulnerable youth, child psychiatrists and other providers should consult and communicate regularly with a multidisciplinary team.[2] Victims often need specialized medical care, mental health counseling, safe housing and guardianship, and legal assistance. Establishing collaborative relationships between providers and outside agencies, such as law enforcement, social workers, and child protective services, encourages a cohesive approach that comprehensively addresses the medical and nonmedical needs of these youth. Indeed, regular professional collaboration constitutes an essential component of treatment of these youth, so much so that child psychiatrists and other mental health professionals who find themselves treating their patients in isolation from other providers and services should recognize that they are not meeting the needs of these patients. Law enforcement, social workers, community and youth advocates (eg, teachers, youth pastors, school counselors, club leaders), and child protective services can all be part of establishing a long-term safety plan for these victims. Shared electronic medical records and confidential email constitutes potentially effective and efficient means of such communication, particularly when many services are involved. Scheduled clinical conferences often provide efficient and effective means of communication and clinical management.

Many states have established specific DMST task forces to address legislative changes (safe harbor laws) and to create a coordinated response once a victim is encountered. Safe harbor laws provide immunity from prosecution and identify specific services for DMST victims.[3] A coordinated response includes consideration of the multifaceted needs of these youth, including housing, family, or social supports; education; safety; and medical and mental health needs. Ideally, participants in the coordinated response appreciate the interconnectedness of these factors. Medical and mental health treatment recommendations are a critical component of court proceedings and overall care coordination. Child and adolescent psychiatrists and mental health providers are, therefore, critical participants in the collaborative process.

Box 1
National resources for domestic minor sex trafficking victims

- Girls Educational and Mentoring Services (GEMS): http://www.gems-girls.org
- Breaking Free: http://www.breakingfree.net/
- National Survivor Network: http://www.castla.org/nsn
- Rehab's Hideaway: http://jointheswitch.org/
- Homeland Security: 1-(800)-973-2867
- Love 146: https://love146.org
- My Life My Choice: http://www.fightingexploitation.org
- National Human Trafficking Resource Center (NHTRC) hotline: 1-(888)-373-7888, http://traffickingresourcecenter.org
- Office for Victims of Crime: http://www.ojp.usdoj.gov/ovc/grants/traffickingmatrix.html
- The National Center for Missing and Exploited Children: 1-(800)-843-5678, http://www.missingkids.org/home

---

Community and National Programs

Providers should be aware of the many community and national level programs and resources available for adolescents at risk or involved in DMST. Many programs offer housing, education, and job opportunities; health services; and survivor mentoring (**Box 1**).

FUTURE DIRECTIONS

The issue of DMST has become increasingly recognized in health care settings; however, there is still a need to continue education, training, and research in the domains of preventative efforts, identification, screening, appropriate interventions, and subsequent resource provision for victimized and high-risk youth. Currently, there are very few evidence-based treatments and programs for survivors of DMST.[45] Additional empirical research and randomized controlled trials addressing intervention options such as TF-CBT specifically for sexually exploited youth in the United States are necessary.

Research should include a needs-assessment of the knowledge gaps, barriers to screening, and clinical decision-making to inform future guidelines addressing acute and follow-up medical care. Furthermore, a standardized national screening tool, ideally implemented in a flexible and discussion-based manner by providers, will improve identification of at-risk and involved youth.

REFERENCES

1. Victims of Trafficking and Violence Protection Act. Available at: http://www.state.gov/j/tip/laws/61124.htm. Accessed June 24, 2016.
2. Greenbaum J, Crawford-Jakubiak J. Child sex trafficking and commercial sexual exploitation: health care needs of victims. Pediatrics 2015;135(3):566–74.
3. Moore JL, Kaplan DM, Barron CE. Sex trafficking of minors. Pediatr Clin North Am 2017;64(2):413–21.
4. Smith LA, Vardaman SH, Snow MA. Domestic minor sex trafficking. Available at: http://sharedhope.org/wp-content/uploads/2012/09/SHI_National_Report_on_DMST_2009.pdf. Accessed December 11, 2015.

5. Muftic LR, Finn MA. Health outcomes among women trafficked for sex in the United States: a closer look. J Interpers Violence 2013;28(9):1859–85.

6. American Professional Society on the Abuse of Children. The commercial sexual exploitation of children: the medical provider's role in identification, assessment and treatment: APSAC practice guidelines. Chicago: APSAC; 2013. Available at: www.kyaap.org/wp-content/uploads/APSAC_Guidelines.pdf. Accessed March 30, 2016.

7. Institute of Medicine and National Research Council. Confronting commercial sexual exploitation and sex trafficking of minors in the United States. Washington, DC: The National Academies Press; 2013.

8. Bryan C. 2014. What judges need to know about human sex trafficking: screening and assessment and matching to empirically based treatment. Presented at the NCJFCJ Annual Conference. Chicago, July 14, 2014.

9. Estes R, Weiner N. The commercial sexual exploitation of children in the U.S., Canada and Mexico. Philadelphia: Center for the Study of Youth Policy, University of Pennsylvania; 2001.

10. Social Ecological Model. Centers for Disease Control and Prevention. 2015. Available at: https://www.cdc.gov/cancer/crccp/sem.htm. Accessed July 7, 2017.

11. Gardner M, Steinberg L. Peer influence on risk taking, risk preference, and risky decision making in adolescence and adulthood: an experimental study. Dev Psychol 2005;41(4):625–35.

12. Goldberg AP, Moore JL, Houck C, et al. Domestic minor sex trafficking patients: a retrospective analysis of medical presentation. J Pediatr Adolesc Gynecol 2017; 30(1):109–15.

13. Stoltz J, Shannon K, Kerr T, et al. Associations between childhood maltreatment and sex work in a cohort of drug-using youth. Soc Sci Med 2007;65(6):1214–21.

14. Steel JL, Herlitz CA. The association between childhood and adolescent sexual abuse and proxies for sexual risk behavior: a random sample of the general population of Sweden. Child Abuse Negl 2005;29(10):1141–53.

15. Chettiar J, Shannon K, Wood E, et al. Survival sex work involvement among street-involved youth who use drugs in a Canadian setting. J Public Health 2010;32:322.

16. Greene JM, Ennett ST, Ringwalt CL. Prevalence and correlates of survival sex among runaway and homeless youth. Am J Public Health 1999;89:1406.

17. Gleghorn AA, Marx R, Vittinghoff E, et al. Association between drug use patterns and HIV risks among homeless, runaway, and street youth in Northern California. Drug Alcohol Depend 1998;51(3):219–27.

18. Edwards JM. Prevalence and correlates of exchanging sex for drugs or money among adolescents in the United States. Sex Transm Infect 2006;82(5):354–8.

19. Moore JL, Houck C, Hirway P, et al. Trafficking experiences and clinical features of domestic minor sex trafficking victims. J Interpers Violence 2017. [Epub ahead of print].

20. Kennedy MA, Klein C, Bristowe JT, et al. Routes of recruitment. J Aggression Maltreat Trauma 2007;15(2):1–19.

21. Wickrama KAS, Diana LB. Adolescent precocious development and young adult health outcomes. Advances in life course research. 2010. Available at: https://www.ncbi.nlm.nih.gov/pmc/articles/PMC3076936/. Accessed July 7, 2017.

22. Kwako L, Noll J, Putnam F, et al. Attachment disorder, sexual behavior problems and sexual abuse. childhood sexual abuse and attachment: an intergenerational perspective. Clin Child Psychol Psychiatry 2011;15(3):169–84.

23. Cobbina JE, Oselin SS. It's not only for the money: an analysis of adolescent versus adult entry into street prostitution. Sociol Inq 2011;81(3):310–32.
24. Leventhal T, Dupéré V, Brooks-Gunn J. Neighborhood influences on adolescent development. In: Handbook of adolescent psychology. New York: John Wiley & Sons, Inc; 2009.
25. Clawson HJ, Dutch N. Addressing the needs of victims of human trafficking: challenges, barriers, and promising practices. Washington, DC: U.S. Department of Health and Human Services, Office of the Assistant Secretary for Planning and Evaluation; 2008. p. 1–10.
26. Egan R, Hawkes G. Endangered girls and incendiary objects: unpacking the discourse on sexualization. Sex Cult 2008;12(4):291–311.
27. Reid JA. An exploratory model of girls vulnerability to commercial sexual exploitation in prostitution. Child Maltreat 2011;16(2):146–57.
28. Adams W, Colleen O, Small K. Effects of federal legislation on the commercial exploitation of children. Juvenile Justice Bulletin. Washington, DC: U.S. Department of Justice, Office of Justice Programs, Office of Juvenile Justice and Delinquency Prevention; 2010. Available at: https://www.ncjrs.gov/pdffiles1/ojjdp/228631.pdf.
29. Curtis R, Terry K, Dank M, et al. The commercial sexual exploitation of children in New York City: Volume 1: the CSEC population in New York City: size, characteristics, and needs [Internet]. Washington, DC: National Institute of Justice, US Department of Justice; 2008. Available at: www.ncjrs.gov/pdffiles1/nij/grants/225083.pdf. Accessed October 2, 2015.
30. Roe-Sepowitz DE, Gallagher J, Risinger M, et al. The sexual exploitation of girls in the United States. J Interpers Violence 2014;30(16):2814–30.
31. Mitchell KJ, Jones LM, Finkelhor D, et al. Internet-facilitated commercial sexual exploitation of children: findings from a nationally representative sample of law enforcement agencies in the United States. Sex Abuse 2010;23(1):43–71.
32. Choo KR. Online child grooming: a literature review on the misuse of social networking sites for grooming children for sexual offenses. Canberra ACT (Australia): Australian Institute of Criminology; 2009.
33. Wells M, Mitchell KJ, Ji K. Exploring the role of the internet in juvenile prostitution Cases coming to the attention of law enforcement. J Child Sex Abus 2012;21(3):327–42.
34. Hopper EK. Psychological coercion and trauma exposure in human trafficking. PsycEXTRA Dataset. http://dx.doi.org/10.1037/e607202010-011.
35. Pence E, Paymar M. Education groups for men who batter. New York: Springer Publishing Company; 1993.
36. Parker SC, Skrmetti JT. Pimps down: a prosecutorial perspective on domestic sex trafficking. University of Memphis Law Review 43. 2013. p. 1013–45.
37. Dutton DG, Painter S. The battered woman syndrome: effects of severity and intermittency of abuse. Am J Orthopsychiatry 1993;63(4):614–22.
38. Lederer L, Wetzel CA. The health consequences of sex trafficking and their implications for identifying victims in healthcare facilities. Ann Health Law 2014;23:61–91.
39. Barron CE, Moore JL, Baird GL, et al. Sex Trafficking Assessment and Resources (STAR) for Pediatric Attendings in Rhode Island. RI Med J 2016;99(9):27–30.
40. Beck M, Lineer M, Melzer-Lange M, et al. Medical providers' understanding of sex trafficking and their experience with at-risk patients. Pediatrics 2015;135(4):e895–902.

41. Titchen KE, Loo D, Berdan E, et al. Domestic sex trafficking of minors: medical student and physician awareness. Pediatr Adolesc Gynecol 2015;30(1):102–8.

42. Ijadi-Maghsoodi R, Cook M, Barnert ES, et al. Understanding and responding to the needs of commercially sexually exploited youth: recommendations for the mental health provider. Child Adolesc Psychiatr Clin N Am 2016;25(1): 107–22.

43. Cohen JA, Mannarino AP, Kinnish K. Trauma-focused cognitive behavioral therapy for commercially sexually exploited youth. J Child Adolesc Trauma 2015; 10(2):175–85.

44. New Index. My Life My Choice. Available at: http://www.fightingexploitation.org/. Accessed July 11, 2017.

45. Felner JK, Dubois DL. Addressing the commercial sexual exploitation of children and youth: a systematic review of program and policy evaluations. J Child Adolesc Trauma 2016;10(2):187–201.

Sports-Related Concussion

Acute Management and Chronic Postconcussive Issues

Navid Mahooti, MD, MPH

KEYWORDS

- Sports-related concussion • Concussion treatment • Vestibular therapy
- Postconcussive syndrome • Return-to-learn • Return-to-play (return-to-sport)
- Neuropsychological testing

KEY POINTS

- Concussion is a functional rather than a structural injury that occurs after a blow to the head or body; standard neuroimaging results are normal and recovery may take up to 4 weeks in children and adolescents under the age of 18 (~10–14 days in adults).
- Cognitive and physical activity modifications are the hallmarks of initial management; prolonged physical and cognitive rest may impede recovery and lead to mood and/or anxiety disorders.
- Athletes with persistent symptoms or postconcussive syndrome should be referred to a vestibular therapist, ideally one with experience or specialty training in concussion management.
- Quality studies supporting pharmacologic treatments are lacking; however, concussion specialists often prescribe various over-the-counter and prescription medications targeting specific symptoms.
- Return-to-learn decisions should precede return-to-sport decisions through the implementation of published, step-wise protocols that are individualized by the clinician according to each student-athlete's particular circumstance, taking into consideration concussion, medical, psychiatric, and any other pertinent history.

INTRODUCTION

It has been said the occurrence and management of sports concussion provokes more debate and concern than virtually all other sports injuries combined.[1] Most concussions are managed by primary care physicians and sports medicine specialists.

Disclosures: The author has no commercial or financial conflicts of interest and no sources of funding to disclose.
North Shore Physicians Group, Mass General/North Shore, 104 Endicott Street Suite 104, Danvers, MA 01923, USA
E-mail address: NMahooti@partners.org

Neurologists and psychiatrists are periodically consulted to aid in the management of athletes with persistent symptoms (postconcussive syndrome). The goal of this article is to highlight issues in sports-related concussion (SRC) that are germane to a practicing child and adolescent psychiatrist. Much of the information herein is gleaned from the 2017 Berlin Consensus Statement on concussion, which is generally considered to be the most authoritative document on SRC.

DEFINITION

According to the 2017 Berlin Consensus Statement on concussion in sport, authored by an international group of interdisciplinary experts known as the Concussion In Sport Group (CISG), "Sport related concussion (SRC) is a traumatic brain injury induced by biomechanical forces… may be caused either by a direct blow to the head, face, neck or elsewhere on the body with an impulsive force transmitted to the head. SRC typically results in the rapid onset of short-lived impairment of neurological function that resolves spontaneously. However, in some cases, signs and symptoms evolve over a number of minutes to hours."[2]

Concussion, often referred to as a mild traumatic brain injury, is a functional disturbance of neurologic function rather than a structural injury, resulting in a wide range of clinical signs and symptoms that typically resolve sequentially and otherwise cannot be explained by substance or medication use, other injuries, or other illnesses. Standard neuroimaging with MRI or computed tomography (CT) is normal. Loss of consciousness (LOC) is relatively uncommon, occurring in about 5% of concussed high school athletes in a descriptive study using an online surveillance program.[3]

EPIDEMIOLOGY

The Centers for Disease Control (CDC) estimates that anywhere from 1.7 to 3.8 million concussions occur in the United States annually. These numbers likely underestimate the true incidence given that athletes underreport. For boys, incidence is highest in football, ice hockey, and wrestling; for girls incidence is highest in soccer, lacrosse, and basketball.[4,5]

PATHOPHYSIOLOGY: NEUROMETABOLIC CASCADE

It is postulated that a concussion results in neuronal disruption that produces a neurometabolic cascade whereby potassium efflux, glutamate release, and lactate accumulation occur, as well as the consequent increased demand for glucose and adenosine triphosphate (ATP), among other factors, in an environment of relatively diminished cerebral blood flow. This supply-demand mismatch is thought to cause concussion symptoms.[6]

DIAGNOSIS

Concussion is a clinical diagnosis whereby the sideline evaluation is based on recognition of injury, assessment of symptoms, cognitive and cranial nerve function, and balance. Serial assessments are often necessary because symptoms may evolve over minutes to hours. The suspected diagnosis of SRC can include 1 or more of the following clinical domains, as described in the Berlin Statement:

1. Symptoms: somatic (eg, headache), cognitive (eg, feeling in a fog), and/or emotional symptoms (eg, lability)
2. Physical signs (eg, LOC, amnesia, neurological deficit)
3. Balance impairment (eg, gait unsteadiness)

4. Behavioral changes (eg, irritability)
5. Cognitive impairment (eg, slowed reaction times)
6. Sleep or wake disturbance (eg, somnolence, drowsiness).

These signs and symptoms are nonspecific, but if one or more are present in the context of an injury to the head or body, concussion should be suspected. The Sports Concussion Assessment Tool, 5th edition (SCAT5; for ages 13 years and older, and Child SCAT5 for ages 5–12 years), is a very helpful tool in guiding the clinician through the initial evaluation of a concussion:

- The SCAT5 or Child SCAT5 (collectively referred to as SCAT) currently represents the most well-established and rigorously developed instrument available for sideline assessment.
- The SCAT is useful immediately after injury in differentiating concussed from non-concussed athletes, but its utility seems to decrease significantly 3 to 5 days after injury.
- The concussion symptom and symptom severity scores, which are part of the SCAT, demonstrate clinical utility in tracking recovery.
- Baseline testing may be useful and, if used, should be performed in the same environment as postconcussion testing. Baseline testing is helpful but not absolutely necessary for interpreting postinjury scores.
- Clinical reaction time, gait or balance assessment, video-observable signs, and oculomotor screening are additional domains that may add to the SCAT.
- Current sensor technology within helmets or attached to headgear or the head itself have limitations in their ability to measure the quality and quantity of head impacts and are of limited clinical use.[2]

RECOVERY

Although most injured athletes recover within the first month of injury, neurobiological recovery might extend beyond clinical recovery in some cases. Psychological factors, such as depression, anxiety, and the feeling of isolation, likely play a significant role in symptom recovery and contribute to the risk of persistent symptoms.[2]

Currently, there is no universally accepted definition of persistent symptoms, also known as postconcussive syndrome. It is generally agreed that concussions in adults age 18 years and older resolve in 10 to 14 days, whereas concussions in youth younger than the age of 18 years may last up to 28 days. Most authorities agree that anything beyond these timeframes is considered persistent. Persistent symptoms do not reflect a single pathophysiological entity but describe a constellation of nonspecific post-traumatic symptoms that may be linked to coexisting and/or confounding factors, which do not necessarily reflect ongoing physiologic injury to the brain. According to the Berlin Statement, "A detailed multimodal clinical assessment is required to identify specific primary and secondary pathologies that may be contributing to persisting post-traumatic symptoms. At a minimum, the assessment should include a comprehensive history, focused physical examination, and special tests where indicated (eg, graded aerobic exercise test). Currently, while there is insufficient evidence for investigations, such as EEG, advanced neuroimaging techniques, genetic testing and biomarkers, to recommend a role in the clinical setting, their use in the research setting is encouraged."[2] **Box 1** and **Table 1** summarize the conclusions of the Berlin Statement with regard to factors that seem to play a role in prolonged clinical recovery.

> **Box 1**
> **Intrinsic factors suspected to play a role in the duration of clinical recovery from sports-related concussion**
>
> - Genetics
> - Sex differences (female more than male gender)
> - Younger age
> - Neurodevelopmental factors (eg, attention deficit hyperactivity disorder or learning disability)
> - Personal or family history of migraine
> - Personal or family history of mental health problems
>
> *Data from* McCrory P, Meeuwisse W, Dvořák J, et al. Consensus statement on concussion in sport—the 5th international conference on concussion in sport held in Berlin, October 2016. Br J Sports Med 2017;51:838–847.

Very little research has been carried out on children younger than the age of 13 years. There is some evidence that high school students might be more vulnerable than other age groups to persistent symptoms, with greater risk for girls than boys.[2]

ADVANCED IMAGING

According to the Zurich Guidelines from 2012 (the predecessor to the Berlin Guidelines), in the acute setting, advanced imaging is recommended if any one of the following is present: LOC longer than 1 minute, progressively worsening symptoms, or a focal neurologic deficit.[7] Most athletes will not meet criteria for neuroimaging. If such symptoms are present acutely, CT of the head is the most readily available imaging modality to rule out intracranial bleeds or structural abnormalities.[8] Given the

Table 1
Likelihood that certain factors suspected to prolong recovery actually do so based on current evidence

Category	Factors	Likelihood
Preinjury individual differences (see **Box 1**)	Personal history of SRC[a]	Likely
Acute or subacute clinical effects and comorbidities	Number and severity of symptoms[b] Initial severity of cognitive deficits Development of post-traumatic headaches or migraines Experiencing dizziness Difficulties with oculomotor functioning Experiencing symptoms of depression	Likely
Initial injury severity indicators	LOC Retrograde amnesia Post-traumatic amnesia	Inconsistent findings

[a] Having multiple past SRCs is associated with having more physical, cognitive, and emotional symptoms before participation in a sporting season.
[b] Strongest and most consistent predictor of slower recovery from SRC.
   Data from McCrory P, Meeuwisse W, Dvořák J, et al. Consensus statement on concussion in sport—the 5th international conference on concussion in sport held in Berlin, October 2016. Br J Sports Med 2017;51:838–847.

potential carcinogenic effects of radiation exposure from CT scans, the risks and benefits should be thoughtfully weighed.[9,10]

In athletes with persistent symptoms, the clinician must use her or his clinical judgment whether to pursue imaging. In an email-based survey by Stache and colleagues[11] of 420 sports medicine physicians (SMPs) that had an 11% responder rate, few respondents (4.5%) reported considering neuroimaging immediately on evaluation, whereas only 2 (0.5%) reported never using neuroimaging in the assessment of concussion. Most indicated that they would consider neuroimaging with an abnormal neurologic examination (85.7%), with worsening symptoms (80.2%), with increased vomiting (69.3%), or with persistent symptoms between 6 and 12 weeks postinjury (51.4%), with an additional 57 respondents (13.6%) who would consider using neuroimaging with persistent symptoms beyond 12 weeks postinjury.

If imaging for persistent symptoms is pursued, MRI is the test of choice because it provides more detailed information and does not expose the patient to ionizing radiation. (Research on other imaging modalities, such as functional MRI, diffusion tensor imaging, and magnetic resonance spectroscopy, is underway but these techniques are not routinely available.) The results are often normal but, occasionally, incidental findings, such as pineal cysts, aneurysms, and Chiari malformations, are encountered. Deciding what to do about these findings can be a real challenge for the ordering physician and downstream consultants who are often asked to weigh in on the matter.[12] These potential quandaries should be considered before imaging. Patient demand, community resources, and physician comfort are common determinants of which patients receive advanced imaging.

NEUROPSYCHOLOGICAL TESTING

Assessment of cognitive function is an important component of concussion management and is a factor in return-to-learn and return-to-play decision-making. The timeframe and extent of the assessment is debatable. No clear evidence-based guidelines are available. The spectrum of options includes the following:

- Pen and paper testing is the gold standard, but testing can take several hours and is often not covered by insurance.
- Computerized neuropsychological (NP) testing is more readily available, less time consuming (~30 minutes), and not as costly, but its routine use and validity have been called into question.[13–15]
- Office-based screening tools, such as the Standardized Assessment of Concussion, which is a part of the SCAT, take about 5 minutes and provide useful cognitive information in the acute and subacute setting, but their applicability in cases of persistent symptoms has not been clearly established.
- Subjective assessment, based on student's self-reported ability to integrate back into class and complete assignments successfully, can also guide clinical decision-making.

NP testing (often called neurocognitive testing) can be a valuable tool in the evaluation and management of concussion. NP testing is not a requirement for all athletes and should not be the sole basis of management decisions. It provides additional information that facilitates clinical decision-making. Ideally, preseason baseline test results (optimally obtained in a similar environment to the follow-up tests) are available for comparison. However, baseline testing is not required; results can be compared with normative data.

When NP testing is used, interpretation is optimally performed by a trained neuro-psychologist in the context of a comprehensive clinical evaluation. In cases in which an athlete reports complete resolution of clinical symptoms yet their computerized NP testing has not returned to baseline (or to age-adjusted norms), return to sport is not necessarily absolutely contraindicated, but caution is advised. In all cases of persistent symptoms, a multidisciplinary team incorporating perspectives from the team physician, primary care physician, psychiatrist, neurologist, vestibular or physical therapist, psychologist, athletic trainer, and whomever else is involved in the athlete's care, is recommended to establish a comprehensive plan of care.

Office-based vestibular and ocular motor screening (VOMS) is a useful examination tool to detect subtle abnormalities (eg, accommodation or convergence deficits) and confirm that recovery is not complete.[16] In a study of 105 healthy adolescents who underwent VOMS testing, the investigators concluded the VOMS did not provoke vestibular symptoms in healthy adolescents and that VOMS items measured unique aspects of vestibular function, other than those measured by the commonly used Balance Error Scoring System (part of the SCAT) and the King-Devick test,[17] with good reliability.[18] VOMS is most commonly performed by vestibular therapists as part of a comprehensive concussion rehabilitation program, but it is also common for sports medicine practitioners to incorporate elements of VOMS into their assessment. No clear guidelines are available to direct clinicians when abnormal VOMS are detected in an otherwise asymptomatic patient who has seemingly recovered. It is prudent to exercise caution with return-to-learn and especially return-to-sport decisions in such patients, and especially useful to have an experienced vestibular therapist who can help interpret and contextualize the VOMS results. A basic understanding of VOMS is recommended for any clinician who cares for patients with concussions.

MANAGEMENT
Acute Symptoms

For years, the mainstay of concussion care has been a common-sense approach of physical and cognitive rest until symptoms improve and then a gradual increase in such activities, as tolerated. However, evidence to support this approach is sparse.[19] In the recent past, based on anecdotal experience, clinicians often recommended complete rest, sometimes referred to as cocooning, for a few days after a concussion. This approach has fallen out of favor because it isolates students and may paradoxically lead to worsening symptoms, namely depression and anxiety. It is now generally advised that after a brief period of rest during the acute phase (24–48 hours) after injury, patients can be encouraged to become gradually and progressively more active while staying below their cognitive and physical symptom-exacerbation thresholds (ie, activity level should not bring on or significantly worsen their symptoms). It is prudent for athletes to avoid vigorous exertion while they are recovering.[2,20]

Tables 2 and 3 summarize the return-to-learn and return-to-sport progression and rationale. Box 2 summarizes the key points in the management of concussions during the acute phase in the pediatric athlete.

Clinicians who care for concussed athletes are assigned the challenging duty of determining whether comorbid conditions, such as chronic migraines, anxiety, post-traumatic stress disorder, attention problems, and sleep dysfunction, are pre-morbid conditions, downstream effects of SRC, or simply associated states, all the while being mindful of the risk of premature return to sport.[2] Moreover, there is potential harm of not allowing a recovered athlete to return to a sport or activity that may make up much of the person's identity and self-worth (especially in elite level athletes). It can be a daunting, unenviable task.

Table 2
Return-to-learn progression and rationale

Stage	Activity	Objective
0	Cognitive rest: no school, no homework, no screen-time Avoid any activities that exacerbate symptoms	Recovery
1	Gradual reintroduction of cognitive activity: ~5–15 min intervals of cognitive activity, as tolerated[a]	Initiate cognitive processes via subsymptom threshold cognitive activities
2	Homework at school before schoolwork at school: homework in ~20–30 min intervals, rest in between	Improve cognitive stamina via repetition of short periods of self-paced cognitive activity
3	School re-entry: once achieved ~1–2 cumulative h/d of homework at home, progress to part-day of school with academic accommodations	Re-entry to school to allow controlled, subsymptom threshold increase in cognitive activities
4	Gradual reintegration into school: wean academic accommodations	Improve cognitive stamina, gain confidence
5	Resumption of full cognitive workload: introduce testing, catch up on essential work	Have fun!

Some students who miss coursework may develop significant anxiety and stress, fearing it may jeopardize their academic standing. Clinicians are wise to assess for these stressors, to reassure the students, and communicate with school officials to facilitate a smooth transition back to the classroom.

[a] To prevent the student from getting too far behind, it is generally recommended that courses with cumulative knowledge (sciences, math) be introduced first.

Adapted from Master CL, Gioia GA, Leddy JJ, et al. Importance of 'return-to-learn' in pediatric and adolescent concussion. Ped Annals 2012;41(9):3; with permission.

In addition to the components found in **Box 2,** The Berlin Statement encourages schools to have an SRC policy that includes education on SRC prevention and management for teachers, staff, students, and parents. Regular medical follow-up after an SRC to monitor recovery and help with return to school is advised, and students may require temporary absence from school after injury. Children and adolescents should not return to sport until they have successfully returned to school.[2] All 50 states have enacted concussion laws with similar requirements, each mandating some type of educational program for clinicians, parents, athletes, and/or all school volunteers. All clinicians are strongly encouraged to learn their state's concussion laws. The CDC's Heads Up Concussion Web site is an excellent resource.

Persistent Symptoms

Treatment of persistent symptoms should be individualized based on a variety of data, including, at the very least, the patient's medical history, concussion history, and psychosocial factors. The Berlin Statement highlights that preliminary evidence supports the following:

1. An individualized symptom-limited aerobic exercise program for patients with persistent postconcussive symptoms associated with autonomic instability or physical deconditioning

Table 3
Return-to-sport progression and rationale

Stage	Activity	Objective
0	Physical rest: avoid any activities that significantly increase symptoms	Recovery
1	Light aerobic activity: walking and swimming Heart rate up to 70% of maximum predicted No resistance training	Increase heart rate
2	Sport-specific exercises: running drills, skating No head impacts	Add movement
3	Noncontact training drills: complex drills. Initiate resistance training	Add cognitive load during exercise, coordination
4	Full contact practice (once cleared by medical professional)	Restore functional skills, confidence, timing, and determine if ready for game-play
5	Return to game play	Have fun!

At stage 0, the athlete typically has symptoms at rest or with light activity.
Adapted from Master CL, Gioia GA, Leddy JJ, et al. Importance of 'return-to-learn' in pediatric and adolescent concussion. Ped Annals 2012;41(9):5; with permission.

2. A targeted physical therapy program in patients with cervical spine or vestibular dysfunction
3. A collaborative approach, including cognitive behavioral therapy, to deal with any persistent mood or behavioral issues.[2]

Moreover, a closely monitored active rehabilitation program incorporating controlled subsymptom-threshold, submaximal exercise, such as the Buffalo Concussion Treadmill Test, has been shown to be safe and may facilitate recovery.[2,21] When chronic

---

Box 2
Key points in the management of pediatric concussions during the acute phase

In a systematic review on concussion in children and adolescents published in the same edition as the Berlin Consensus Statement, Davis and colleagues drew the following conclusions based on the available literature.

- Child and adolescent age-specific paradigms should be applied.
- Child-validated symptom rating scales should be used.
- The expected duration of symptoms associated with SRC is less than 4 weeks.
- Prolonged recovery is defined as symptomatic for longer than 4 weeks.
- A brief period of cognitive and physical rest should be followed with gradual symptom-limited physical and cognitive activity.
- All schools be encouraged to have a concussion policy and should offer appropriate academic. Accommodations and support to students recovering from SRC.
- Children and adolescents should not return to sport until they have successfully returned to school. Early introduction of symptom-limited physical activity is appropriate.

From Davis GA, Anderson V, Babl FE, et al. What is the difference in concussion management in children as compared with adults? A systematic review. Br J Sports Med 2017;51:949–57; with permission.

postconcussive symptoms are triggered exclusively by academic work or school attendance but not by physical activity, other factors, such as an underlying anxiety disorder, should be considered.

Cervicogenic headaches in particular and concussions in general can be effectively treated with traditional psychotherapy,[22] physical and vestibular therapy, myofascial release or massage, greater occipital nerve blocks, biofeedback, or trigger point injections.[23,24] Hyperbaric oxygen therapy (HBOT) has been used as well,[25] but a recent literature review of 5 level 1 studies concluded there is more evidence to refute the use of HBOT for postconcussion syndrome than to support it.[26] The anecdotal benefits of craniosacral therapy and osteopathic manipulation therapy are prevalent on the Internet, but there is a dearth of evidence in the literature to support these modalities.

PHARMACOTHERAPY

Although no medications are currently approved by the US Food and Drug Administration for the treatment of a sport-related concussion, many supplements, as well as over-the-counter and prescription medications, have been used to reduce headaches, improve sleep, improve cognitive function, and address psychological comorbidities associated with concussion. In a survey of pediatricians, most respondents (89%) managed the symptoms of concussed patients with medications, most commonly acetaminophen (62%) or nonsteroidal anti-inflammatory medications (NSAIDs) (54%). The use of prescription medications, such as tricyclic antidepressants (23%), amantadine (10%), and methylphenidate (8%), was also commonly reported. Pediatricians treating more than 16 patients per year with concussion were more likely to prescribe tricyclic antidepressants, stimulants, and agents used for sleep disturbance, and less likely to prescribe NSAIDs. Other commonly used medications were melatonin (20%), tricyclic antidepressants (20%), amantadine (10%), and stimulants (8%).[27] In a similar survey of pediatric emergency medicine physicians, acetaminophen was used by 78% and NSAIDs by 77%. Ondansetron was also used frequently (54%), with narcotic use to a much lesser extent (7%).[28] In the Stache and colleagues[11] survey of SMPs, 47.9% of respondents (compared with 89% of pediatricians) indicated they use medication to treat concussion symptoms within the first 48 hours postinjury; 76% reported using medication to treat concussion symptoms beyond 48 hours postinjury.[11] A review of specific pharmacotherapies for postconcussive symptoms and associated comorbidities follows.

Supplements

A variety of supplements, including omega 3 fatty acids (O3FAs), magnesium, B vitamins, curcumin, green tea, resveratrol, creatine, vitamin C, vitamin D, and vitamin E, and *Scutellaria baicalensis*, as well as various diets and foods, are used and often recommended by clinicians. O3FAs are probably the most commonly used supplement for the treatment of concussion. Eicosapentaenoic acid and docosahexaenoic acid (DHA) have shown promising neuroprotective properties in animal studies: supplementation with O3FA in rats before sustaining a concussion can protect against reduced plasticity of neurons and impaired learning by normalizing levels of proteins associated with neuronal circuit function, cognitive processing, synaptic facilitation, neuronal excitability, and locomotor control.[29] Supplementation with O3FA after sustaining a concussion can also help maintain genomic stability and cellular homeostasis,[30] as well as decrease the amount of injury the brain sustains.[31] DHA supplementation has been shown to significantly reduce the number of swollen, disconnected, and injured axons when administered following traumatic brain injury.[32] No high-level human studies have been performed to confirm these animal findings.[33]

General Approach: Symptom Clusters

As outlined in **Box 3**, some authorities posit that medications should not be routinely administered unless certain conditions are met. If pharmacotherapy is considered for persistent symptoms, the criteria delineated in **Box 3** should be met.

SRC specialists often categorize the 22 established concussion symptoms into 4 clusters: physical (mostly headache), cognitive, emotional, and sleep disturbance, as noted in **Table 4**. Clustering allows the clinician to identify the most burdensome symptoms and direct therapeutic options accordingly.[34,35]

HEADACHES OR SOMATIC SYMPTOMS
Analgesics

A retrospective chart review at a headache clinic found that 70.1% of adolescent patients with chronic posttraumatic headaches met International Headache Society criteria for probable medication-overuse headaches. Once the culprit over-the-counter medications (NSAIDs, acetaminophen) were discontinued, 68.5% of the patients reported return to their baseline preconcussion headache status. The investigators concluded that excessive use of analgesics postconcussion may contribute to chronic post-traumatic headaches in some adolescents. Management of patients with chronic post-traumatic headache should include analgesic detoxification when medication overuse is suspected.[38]

Amitriptyline

Amitriptyline is often prescribed for postconcussive headaches, and its sedative effects make it an ideal medication in patients with comorbid sleep disturbance. It may also provide antidepressant effects. β-blockers, calcium channel blockers, valproic acid, topiramate, triptans, dihydroergotamine, and gabapentin have all been discussed as potential medical therapies for persistent headaches after concussion and may make reasonable choices in the appropriate circumstances.[34]

COGNITIVE SYMPTOMS
Amantadine

In a retrospective, case-control study of 25 age, sex, and concussion-history matched adolescent boys and girls, the treatment group received 100 mg of amantadine twice daily (200 mg total per day) following a period of rest. Matched controls were evaluated and treated conservatively without medication at the same concussion program

---

Box 3
Three conditions that should be met before a trial of medication is prescribed

1. The athlete's symptoms have exceeded the typical recovery period for a SRC.

2. The symptoms are negatively affecting the patient's life to such a degree that the possible benefit of treatment outweighs the potential risks of the medication being considered.

3. The clinician caring for the athlete is knowledgeable and experienced in the assessment and management of SRC or concussive brain injury in general.

From Meehan WP. Medical therapies for concussion. Clin Sports Med 2011;30(1):117; with permission.

Table 4
The 22 symptoms on the Sports Concussion Assessment Tool, 5th edition, subdivided into 4 clusters to facilitate targeted treatment

Cluster	Physical	Cognitive	Emotional	Sleep

Symptoms	Headaches
	Head pressure
	Neck pain
	Nausea or vomiting
	Dizziness
	Blurry vision
	Balance problems
	Light sensitivity
	Noise sensitivity
		Feeling slowed
		  down
		Feeling in a fog
		Do not feel right
		Concentration
		  difficulties
		Memory difficulties
		Fatigue or low
		  energy
		Confusion
		Drowsiness
			More emotional
			More irritable
			Sadness
			Nervous or
			  anxious
				Trouble
				  falling
				  asleep

Treatment Options (symptom-directed)	Headache
	  prophylaxis
	• Amitriptyline
	• Beta blockers
	• Calcium channel
	  blockers
	Antinausea (acute
	  phase)
	• Ondansetron
		Neurostimulants
		• Amantadine
		• Methylphenidate
		• Atomoxetine
			Selective
			  serotonin
			  reuptake
			  inhibitors
			Trazodone
			Neurostimulants
			Amitriptyline
				Melatonin
				Trazodone[a]

[a] Commonly used in adult medicine for insomnia[36]; data for its use in the pediatric population are nearly nonexistent.[37]

before the start of the amantadine protocol. In this small study of 50 adolescents who underwent computerized neurocognitive testing, amantadine seemed to be an effective pharmacologic treatment of certain concussion-related cognitive deficits and symptoms in athletes with protracted recovery of more than 3 weeks.[39]

Methylphenidate

Methylphenidate acts as a stimulant to help improve cognitive function. Several studies exist in the literature evaluating the use of methylphenidate for improving cognition and mental fatigue after traumatic brain injury. These studies tend to focus on adults, and those that evaluate pediatric-aged patients are often small in number or focus on patients with moderate to severe traumatic brain injuries. To date, no research trials have been published regarding the use of methylphenidate or other similar stimulants in the use of a pediatric sports concussion.

EMOTIONAL SYMPTOMS
Selective Serotonin Reuptake Inhibitors

There are few data to guide clinicians regarding the role of selective serotonin reuptake inhibitors, and no known research studies have been published on the use of the nonselective serotonin reuptake inhibitor trazodone for sleep disturbances after pediatric concussion.[40] In a 2005 study to investigate the effects of methylphenidate and sertraline compared with placebo on various neuropsychiatric sequelae associated with mild to moderate traumatic brain injury, methylphenidate and sertraline had similar effects on depressive symptoms. However, methylphenidate seemed to be more beneficial in improving cognitive function and maintaining daytime alertness. Methylphenidate was also better tolerated than sertraline.[41] Despite this lack of data, the survey by Stache and colleagues[11] revealed that 24% of SMPs prescribe either trazodone or a selective serotonin reuptake inhibitor in patients who have symptoms beyond 48 hours. These medications may be beneficial, but some authorities recommend that depressive symptoms are best handled by a psychiatrist (and/or pediatrician) who will be following the patient longer-term.[34]

SLEEP DISTURBANCE
Sleep Hygiene

Management of sleep disturbance should probably begin with a discussion about the importance of sleep hygiene.[34,42]

Melatonin

Melatonin is often used as an over-the-counter sleep aid. Its safety profile makes it an excellent candidate for assisting with sleep. It may also have other beneficial roles in recovery from traumatic brain injury.[43] These neuroprotective effects have not been studied in actual human models; no published research exists regarding melatonin use for concussions. An ongoing double-blind, placebo-controlled randomized trial is examining the use of melatonin in children with postconcussive sleep disturbance.[33,44]

PHARMACOTHERAPY: BOTTOM LINE

Evidence to support the use of pharmacotherapy is limited.[11] If introduced, almost all SMPs (84%) thought the medication should be discontinued before allowing athletes to return to sports or vigorous physical activity. The return-to-sport decision must be considered with extreme caution while the athlete is on any medications that may mask or modify the symptoms of SRC. Such cases are challenging and should be managed in a multidisciplinary, collaborative setting by health care providers with experience in SRC.

RETIREMENT FROM SPORTS

Retirement from sport is a complex, challenging decision for athletes, physicians, and family members, among others. A conservative approach using a multidisciplinary team is generally advocated. Readers with interest in this topic are referred to an article by Ellis and colleagues,[45] who shared their experiences and evolving multidisciplinary institutional approach to decision-making in this area.

PREVENTION STRATEGIES

Over the past decade, the sports medicine community has witnessed an explosion in concussion prevention strategies. Concussion-prevention strategies can reduce the number and severity of concussions in many sports.

Despite many studies examining SRC-prevention interventions across several sports, some findings remain inconclusive because of conflicting evidence, lack of rigorous study design, and inherent study biases. Additional well-designed studies are needed.[2] Readers with interest in this topic are directed to the Berlin Statement.

THE FUTURE

A recent systematic review by McCrea and colleagues[46] concludes, "Advanced neuroimaging, fluid biomarkers and genetic testing are important research tools, but require further validation to determine their ultimate clinical utility in the evaluation of SRC. Future research efforts should address current gaps that limit clinical translation."

SUMMARY POINTS

- Concussion is a clinical diagnosis based on recognition of injury, assessment of symptoms, cognitive and cranial nerve function, and balance. Serial assessments are often necessary because symptoms may evolve over time, especially in the acute phase.
- Although it is generally agreed that concussion symptoms in youth younger than 18 years may last up to 28 days, currently no definition of persistent symptoms, also known as postconcussive syndrome, in youth or adults, is universally accepted.
- Persistent symptoms do not reflect a single pathophysiological entity but describe a constellation of nonspecific post-traumatic symptoms that may relate to coexisting and/or confounding factors, which do not necessarily reflect ongoing physiologic injury to the brain.
- The science of SRC is imperfect. Individual management and return-to-play decisions remain in the realm of clinical judgment and, whenever possible or necessary, guided by a multidisciplinary team.
- Evidence supporting the use of pharmacotherapeutic agents is limited and largely based on expert opinion but does seem to improve some symptoms.
- Clinicians caring for athletes with SRC should be familiar with the Berlin Consensus guidelines document, the accompanying SCAT5 and Child SCAT5 clinical assessment tools (freely available), and state concussion laws. The CDC's Heads Up Web site is an excellent resource.
- Return-to-learn and, especially, return-to-sport decisions should be individualized. Children and adolescents should not return to sport until they have successfully returned to school. When chronic postconcussive symptoms are triggered exclusively by academic work or school attendance but not by physical activity, other potential psychiatric factors should be considered.

REFERENCES

1. McCrory P. Future advances and areas of future focus in the treatment of sport-related concussion. Clin Sports Med 2011;30(1):201–8, xi–ii.
2. McCrory P, Meeuwisse W, Dvořák J, et al. Consensus statement on concussion in sport—the 5th international conference on concussion in sport held in Berlin, October 2016. Br J Sports Med 2017;51:838–47.
3. Meehan W, d'Hemecourt P, Comstock RD. High school concussions in the 2008-2009 academic year: mechanism, symptoms, and management. Am J Sports Med 2010;38(12):2405–9.
4. Marar M, McIlvain NM, Fields SK, et al. Epidemiology of concussions among United States high school athletes in 20 sports. Am J Sports Med 2012;40(4): 747–55.
5. Lincoln AE, Caswell SV, Almquist JL, et al. Trends in concussion incidence in high school sports: a prospective 11-year study. Am J Sports Med 2011;39(5):958–63.
6. Giza CC, Hovda DA. The new neurometabolic cascade of concussion. Neurosurgery 2014;75(Suppl 4):S24–33.

7. McCrory P, Meeuwisse WH, Aubry M, et al. Consensus statement on concussion in sport: the 4th international conference on concussion in sport held in Zurich, 2012. Br J Sports Med 2013;(47):250–8.

8. Eierud C, Craddock RC, Fletcher S, et al. Neuroimaging after mild traumatic brain injury: review and meta-analysis. Neuroimage Clin 2014;4:283–94.

9. Brenner DJ, Hall EJ. Computed tomography — an increasing source of radiation exposure. N Engl J Med 2007;357:2277–84.

10. Pearce MS, Salotti JA, Little MP, et al. Radiation exposure from CT scans in childhood and subsequent risk of leukaemia and brain tumours: a retrospective cohort study. Lancet 2012;380(9840):499–505.

11. Stache S, Howell D, Meehan WP 3rd. Concussion management practice patterns among sports medicine physicians. Clin J Sport Med 2016;26(5):381–5.

12. Anderson, Pauline. Incidental MRI findings in children on the rise. 2015. Available at: http://www.medscape.com/viewarticle/842893. Accessed June 4, 2017.

13. Schatz P, Moser RS, Solomon GS, et al. Prevalence of invalid computerized baseline neurocognitive test results in high school and collegiate athletes. J Athl Train 2012;47(3):289–96.

14. Arrieux, Jacques P et al. A review of the validity of computerized neurocognitive assessment tools in mild traumatic brain injury assessment. 2017. Available at: http://www.futuremedicine.com/doi/full/10.2217/cnc-2016-0021. Accessed June 6, 2017.

15. Scorza KA, Raleigh MF, O'Connor FG. Current concepts in concussion: evaluation and management. Am Fam Physician 2012;85(2):123–32.

16. Mucha A, Collins MW, Elbin RJ, et al. A brief vestibular/ocular motor screening (VOMS) assessment to evaluate concussions. Am J Sports Med 2014;42(10): 2479–86.

17. Galetta KM, Barrett J, Allen M, et al. The King-Devick test as a determinant of head trauma and concussion in boxers and MMA fighters. Neurology 2011; 76(17):1456–62.

18. Yorke AM, Smith L, Babcock M, et al. Validity and reliability of the vestibular/ ocular motor screening and associations with common concussion screening tools. Sports Health 2016;9(2):174–80.

19. McLeod TC, Lewis JH, Whelihan K, et al. Rest and return to activity after sport-related concussion: a systematic review of the literature. J Athl Train 2017;52(3):262–87.

20. Stelzik J. The role of active recovery and "rest" after concussion. Pediatr Ann 2017;46(4):e139–44.

21. Leddy JJ, Willer B. Use of graded exercise testing in concussion and return-to-activity management. Curr Sports Med Rep 2013;12(6):370–6.

22. Packard RC. Epidemiology and pathogenesis of posttraumatic headache. J Head Trauma Rehabil 1999;14:9–21.

23. Zaremski JL, Herman DC, Clugston JR, et al. Occipital neuralgia as a sequela of sports concussion: a case series and review of the literature. Curr Sports Med Rep 2015;14(1):16–9.

24. Kennedy E, Quinn D, Tumilty S, et al. Clinical characteristics and outcomes of treatment of the cervical spine in patients with persistent post-concussion symptoms: a retrospective analysis. Musculoskelet Sci Pract 2017;29:91–8.

25. Wolf G, Cifu D, Baugh L, et al. The effect of hyperbaric oxygen on symptoms after mild traumatic brain injury. J Neurotrauma 2012;29:2606–12.

26. Hawkins JR, Gonzalez KE, Heumann KJ. The effectiveness of hyperbaric oxygen therapy as a treatment for postconcussion symptoms. J Sport Rehabil 2017; 26(3):290–4.

27. Kinnaman KA, Mannix RC, Comstock RD, et al. 3rd Management strategies and medication use for treating paediatric patients with concussions. Acta Paediatr 2013;102:e424–8.

28. Kinnaman KA, Mannix RC, Comstock RD, et al. Management of pediatric patients with concussion by emergency medicine physicians. Pediatr Emerg Care 2014; 30:458–61.

29. Wu A, Ying Z, Gomez-Pinilla F. Dietary omega-3 fatty acids normalize BDNF levels, reduce oxidative damage, and counteract learning disability after traumatic brain injury in rats. J Neurotrauma 2004;21:1457–67.

30. Wu A, Ying Z, Gomez-Pinilla F. Omega-3 fatty acids supplementation restores mechanisms that maintain brain homeostasis in traumatic brain injury. J Neurotrauma 2007;24:1587–95.

31. Bailes JE, Mills JD. Docosahexaenoic acid reduces traumatic axonal injury in a rodent head injury model. J Neurotrauma 2010;27:1617–24.

32. Petraglia AL, Winkler EA, Bailes JE. Stuck at the bench: potential natural neuroprotective compounds for concussion. Surg Neurol Int 2011;2:146.

33. Ashbaugh A, McGrew C. The role of nutritional supplements in sports concussion treatment. Curr Sports Med Rep 2016;15(1):16–9.

34. Meehan WP. Medical therapies for concussion. Clin Sports Med 2011;30(1): 115–24, ix.

35. Reddy CC. A treatment paradigm for sports concussion. Brain Inj Prof 2004;4: 24–5.

36. Generali JA, Cada DJ. Trazodone: insomnia (adults). Hosp Pharm 2015;50(5): 367–9.

37. El-Chammas K, Keyes J, Thompson N, et al. A comparative effectiveness meta-analysis of drugs for the prophylaxis of pediatric migraine headache. JAMA Pediatr 2013;167(3):250–8.

38. Heyer GL, Idris SA. Does analgesic overuse contribute to chronic post-traumatic headache in adolescent concussion patients? Pediatr Neurol 2014;50:464–8.

39. Reddy CC, Collins M, Lovell M, et al. Efficacy of amantadine on symptoms and neurocognitive performance among adolescents following sports-related concussion. J Head Trauma Rehabil 2013;28:260–5.

40. Halstead ME. Pharmacologic therapies for pediatric concussions. Sports Health 2016;8(1):50–2.

41. Lee H. Comparing effects of methylphenidate, sertraline and placebo on neuropsychiatric sequelae in patients with traumatic brain injury. Hum Psychopharmacol 2005;20(2):97–104.

42. Rao V, Rollings P. Sleep disturbances following traumatic brain injury. Curr Treat Options Neurol 2002;4:77–87.

43. Maldonado MD, Murillo-Cabezas F, Terron MP, et al. The potential of melatonin in reducing morbidity-mortality after craniocerebral trauma. J Pineal Res 2007; 42:1–11.

44. Barlow KM, Brooks BL, MacMaster FP, et al. A double-blind, placebo-controlled intervention trial of 3 and 10 mg sublingual melatonin for post-concussion syndrome in youths (PLAYGAME): study protocol for a randomized controlled trial. Trials 2014;15:271.

45. Ellis MJ, McDonald PJ, Cordingley D, et al. Retirement-from-sport considerations following pediatric sports-related concussion: case illustrations and institutional approach. Neurosurg Focus 2016;40(4):E8.
46. McCrea M, Meier T, Huber D, et al. Role of advanced neuroimaging, fluid bio-markers and genetic testing in the assessment of sport-related concussion: a systematic review. Br J Sports Med 2017;51(12):919–29.

Everywhere and Nowhere

Grief in Child and Adolescent Psychiatry and Pediatric Clinical Populations

Pamela J. Mosher, MD, MDiv[a,b,c,*]

KEYWORDS

• Grief • Child • Adolescent • Psychiatry • Pediatric • Illness

KEY POINTS

- Grief is ubiquitous in the experience of children and adolescents with illness but not always recognized or named, and as a result grief is not always treated effectively by child/adolescent psychiatrists or pediatricians.
- Grief can be misinterpreted or treated as stress, anxiety, depression, adolescent moodiness, or behavioral concerns.
- Pediatricians and child/adolescent psychiatrists are often insufficiently educated on the topic of grief.

In her foreword to the book, *On Grief and Grieving*, by Elizabeth Kübler-Ross and David Kessler, Maria Shriver wrote, "we are a grief-illiterate nation" and "we live in a culture that doesn't know how to grieve."[1] Western societies have been criticized for struggling with death and bereavement generally, leading to a "public absence/private presence of death."[2] Discussing the death of her husband, Facebook executive Sheryl Sandberg said that grief taught her, "I got it all wrong before. I used to say, 'Is there anything I can do?' I used to say, 'How are you?' or not say anything. Every mistake that someone else made with me, I've made."[3] Why is the culture illiterate with respect to grief? Why do compassionate, thoughtful adults not know what to say when someone nearby is grieving? If this criticism holds for society at large, with adults often ill-equipped to navigate grief, what does this mean for children and adolescents? The purpose of this article is to

No conflicts of interest.
^a Division of Child and Adolescent Psychiatry, Hospital for Sick Children, Toronto, ON, Canada;
^b Division of Psychosocial Oncology, Princess Margaret Cancer Centre, Toronto, ON, Canada;
^c Department of Psychiatry, University of Toronto, Toronto, ON, Canada
* Division of Child and Adolescent Psychiatry, Hospital for Sick Children, 555 University Avenue, 1st Floor Burton Wing, Toronto, ON M5G 1X8, Canada
E-mail addresses: pamela.mosher@uhn.ca; pamela.mosher@sickkids.ca

Child Adolesc Psychiatric Clin N Am 27 (2018) 109–124
http://dx.doi.org/10.1016/j.chc.2017.08.009
1056-4993/18/© 2017 Elsevier Inc. All rights reserved.

review basic types of grief and discuss how psychiatrists and other clinicians can support grieving youth.

The death of a loved one engenders perhaps the most recognized form of grief that children and adolescents experience—often seen as devastating, disruptive, and outside the natural order of childhood experience (eg, parental or sibling death). Additional losses leading to grief in children and adolescents with medical and/or psychological illnesses are discussed. Curiously, grief is a topic that does not appear in medical education, or in the child and adolescent psychiatry literature, as often as might be beneficial to our clinical work. If child/adolescent psychiatrists remain mindful of the decentering potential of grief in the lives of young people, they can assist patients more ably through this process, decrease isolation, and reduce the impact of comorbidities associated with grief in childhood.

National statistics and studies regarding the prevalence of childhood and adolescent grief are limited and vary in estimates, and some although oft-quoted sources are now outdated. Yet overall, extant sources reveal that grief often touches the lives of children and adolescents. US Census Bureau data have shown that 1 in 20 children under age 15 years has experienced the death of 1 or both biological parents.[4] As high as 92% of adolescents and young adults in 1 UK study had experienced grief from the death of a "close" or "significant" relationship.[2] In another, 78% of children aged 11 years to 16 years reported experiencing the death of a close friend or relative.[5] Approximately 70,000 to 75,000 children die each year in the United States, and more than 80% of them have siblings who must live with this primary loss.[6] Additionally, 1 to 2 million American children live in single-parent households as a result of a parent's death.[7] A recent longitudinal study of 7 million people in Scandinavia revealed that youth suffering parental death prior to age 18 remain at increased risk for suicide "for at least 25 years," and the risk for men is twice that of women.[8] In addition, adults who experienced parental loss as children have 50% higher all-cause mortality rates and die earlier than same-aged adults with living parents.[9]

In 2012 the American Federation of Teachers and New York Life Foundation[10] undertook a national childhood bereavement survey of schoolteachers; 70% of teachers knew at least 1 student who lost a parent, guardian, sibling, or friend in the past year, whereas only 1% received bereavement training in university or graduate school. The impact of grief noted by teachers included: 87% reported grieving students with impaired classroom concentration, 82% observed withdrawal/disengagement and decreased classroom participation, 79% noticed depression/sadness in students, 72% documented student absenteeism postloss, 68% reported lower quality of schoolwork with 66% noting a decrease in homework submission, and 63% observed anger in grieving students—78% of teachers were unaware of any community bereavement supports.[10]

Given such evidence and the lack of bereavement training among teachers, social workers, and other frontline professionals,[7] child and adolescent psychiatrists have an essential role in grief education and clinical practice, and must remain cognizant that grief has the potential to appear anywhere in the lives of children and adolescents, and grieving youth require unique supports.

Grief is not limited to the experience after another person's death, and clinicians must consider the range of losses that create grief for a child or adolescent. Grief follows diverse losses, including deaths of pets; loss of intact families through separation or divorce; loss of home, neighborhood, friends, and school through moving; loss through adoption or foster care; and loss of loved ones to homelessness, addiction, or incarceration. For youth with medical illnesses, grief can be ubiquitous, emerging from various deficits and constraints that illness imposes on their bodies and life trajectories. For youth with combined physical and mental health issues, such losses can disrupt multiple domains of life, including physical, social, psychological, educational, familial, and existential, among others. When clinicians recognize that grief arises from differing losses, grief becomes more visible in the lives of youth with illness. For children with chronic or life-limiting illness (medical or psychiatric), the following losses, among others, may occur:

- Loss of connection with school, peers, family, or pets, due to symptoms, prolonged treatment, and/or hospital admissions
- Loss of participation in cherished activities (sports, music, and art)
- Loss of physical capacity, bodily integrity, or prior appearance
- Disruption to developmental trajectories in social, educational, home, and physical spheres
- Loss of personal identity, self-concept, self-esteem, resilience, hope, even stable mood or behavior

Prevalent themes among grieving youth are that their experiences or emotions are not acknowledged, they feel different from peers, and that they often find there is nowhere to discuss their feelings.[2] Children and adolescents may not know peers with similar experiences. Without spaces in which to process and integrate their losses with informed adults or grieving peers, young people may feel confused, guilty, or alone and may miss opportunities for culturally accepted grief support. Thus, although grief may be nearly everywhere for young people, it may also feel to them that it is nowhere—particularly given limited societal grief literacy.

Despite the prevalence and diversity of grief, it remains the case in North American medical education that little time is dedicated to training physicians in the diagnosis or management of grief in adult patients, let alone pediatric patients. Given grief's broad reach, increased dialogue among child and adolescent psychiatrists, primary clinicians, and interprofessional colleagues is critical to bring child/adolescent grief more into the collective professional consciousness and daily clinical care.

THEORIES AND MODELS OF GRIEF: STAGES VERSUS TASKS

The psychiatrist Elizabeth Kübler-Ross made famous the concept of traditional, ordered stages of grieving (denial, anger, bargaining, depression, and acceptance). In recent decades, however, the field has evolved from this 5-stage model to a set of theories where those grieving must eventually navigate tasks of grief. Well known examples include Worden's[11] 4 tasks of mourning or grieving, Wolfelt's[12] 6 needs of mourning, and Rando's[13] 6 R processes of mourning. Children move through these tasks at different rates, in different order, and over variable periods of time.[14] Worden's classic tasks of mourning for children and adolescents include the following[11]:

1. "Accepting the reality of the loss (according to the developmental stage/age of the child)
2. Working through the pain and emotional aspects of grief
3. Adjusting to an environment in which the deceased is missing
4. Finding ways to relocate the deceased person within one's life and to memorialize the person"

Many youth find their way through these tasks without requiring professional support, whereas a subset need guidance from clinicians to navigate grief's complex landscape. Psychiatrists may encounter either group clinically, thus defining terms and reviewing types of grief is useful.

DEFINITION OF TERMS
Bereavement

The state of having experienced a loss through death (not the response to such a loss).[15]

Mourning

"The array of psychological processes set in motion by the loss to facilitate adaptation"[16] or, "the outward expression of [one's] thoughts and feelings."[12]

Grief

"Intense sorrow, especially caused by someone's death." (Oxford English Dictionary) "The psychobiological response to bereavement."[16]

The "psychological, behavioral, social, and physical reactions to the perception of loss."[13]

Importantly, grief is unique to individuals and no 2 grieve in a similar fashion; thus, people in 1 family grieving the same loss grieve differently. Because grief experiences are sundry, there is no single way to grieve, and terms such as *normal* or *ordinary*, although used in the past, are now often avoided. The term *typical grief* is used by some contemporary writers to capture this concept.

Acute Grief

"The initial response, often intense and disruptive, to a loss."[16]

A "definite syndrome with psychological and somatic symptomatology."[17]

Acute grief occurs in the immediate aftermath of the loss but is often present for several months.

Integrated Grief

"The permanent response after adaptation to the loss, in which satisfaction in ongoing life is renewed."[16] The reality of death has been incorporated into life, and one begins to return to active, meaningful participation in a changed life.[18] Research indicates that typically within 6 to 12 months, many people transition through acute grief to more integrated grief, although this can take longer.

Uncomplicated Grief

Grief experienced after the death of an important person (called "typical" grief by some investigators),[14] which often becomes integrated grief 6 months to 12 months later.

Grief is never a linear experience internally—it is unpredictable, with significant ebbing and flowing for adults, children, and youth. This unpredictability and the attendant jumble of feelings and physical symptoms experienced can be confusing for youth. The following is a list of potential symptoms and signs that children and adolescents may manifest during grief.

Emotional signs/symptoms of grief
• Sadness, with or without crying
• Anger, with or without aggression
• Guilt, blame
• Fearfulness (of being/sleeping alone, or of other family members dying from accident or illness)

- Anxiety (eg, for others' physical health and safety)
- Irritability
- Confusion
- A jumble/mix of emotions, difficult to describe or distinguish one from another
- Loneliness, isolation, feeling different from peers
- Low frustration tolerance
- Feeling overwhelmed
- Feeling of going crazy
- Disbelief, denial
- Amotivation
- Ruminating/preoccupation about the death or deceased person
- Yearning to be with the deceased person (common, different entity from active suicidal ideation, must not be pathologized)
- Silliness
- Oppositionality or defiance
- Believing everything is fine

Physical symptoms or behaviors of grief

- Fatigue
- Difficulty with concentration, focus, attention, memory (especially at school)
- Speaking rarely or frequently about deceased
- Insomnia, hypersomnia
- Increased or decreased appetite
- Nausea, abdominal discomfort, diarrhea, gastrointestinal upset
- Somatic complaints (headaches, pain, drop attacks, and so forth)
- Regression
  - Bladder/bowel incontinence
  - Sleeping with parents
  - Thumb-sucking
  - Speaking in baby voice
  - Separation anxiety
- Aggressive outbursts at any age (or angry play in younger children)
- Nightmares
- Withdrawal from family/friends
- Imitation of deceased person
- Restlessness
- Behaving as if everything is fine
- Decline in school performance; school avoidance
- Substance use (drugs, alcohol, and so forth)
- Self-injurious behavior
- Other high-risk behaviors

GRIEF AND DEVELOPMENTAL STAGES

Young children, school-aged children, preteens, and adolescents grieve differently according to their different cognitive and emotional developmental stages, and this can confuse adults around them. What follows is a brief introduction to grief and developmental stages.

Bowlby,[19,20] and others describe infants detecting caregiver absences, so routines should be maintained as much as possible when a parent or caregiver dies. Preschool children do not yet comprehend death as permanent. Believing it is temporary, they often ask if the deceased is still eating, walking, or sleeping or when the deceased will be returning. Again, routines and schedules are to be maintained as much as possible with familiar caregivers. Younger children typically grieve in bursts or doses, for example, embarking on death-related play during the funeral or social gatherings after a death. They may halt play, ask a trusted adult detailed questions about the death, and then swiftly return to other play and laughter. This is normal grief behavior for young children and should be understood in developmental context and not pathologized. Magical thinking characterizes this age—children may believe they caused the death or are somehow to blame for their thoughts, words, or deeds. Younger children do not possess comprehensive language or understanding for the emotions of grief, and this can lead to palpable confusion, loss of control, and acting out. Adults can help by providing age-appropriate details about illness, death, funerals, and so forth, in small doses, with concrete explanations. They can show by example it is okay to cry and talk about and remember the deceased in various ways over time.

Schoolchildren may focus more on their own needs and concerns than on the deceased. They may ask questions about who will put them to bed, take them to school, make lunches, or drive them to lessons or games in lieu of the deceased. School-aged children begin to understand death's finality and may focus on the surviving parent/caregivers, worrying significantly about their health or potential death. They often ask specific, scientific questions about death, what happens to the body once buried, and so forth. They may still hold magical thoughts, believing they somehow caused the death, which may induce regret, fear, and self-blame. It is essential to reassure children the death is not their fault. Adults can provide consistency, reassurance, and honest, developmentally-appropriate answers to this age group.

For adolescents in Western cultures, it is developmentally appropriate to process feelings, thoughts, and stressors with peers, not parents. It may be unrealistic, therefore, to expect a teenager to discuss grief or death with a parent. Adolescents and children wish to appear normal, and grief marks them as different from peers, thus underscoring their yearning. They may be unwilling or unable to discuss grief with any peer inexperienced with it, which can lead to a double sense of isolation for adolescents. Externalizing and internalizing tendencies may drive risk-taking behaviors, substance use, changes in personality and school performance, and so forth. Piaget's formal operations stage affords adolescents the capacity for existential and abstract thought, thus increasingly adult approaches to grief.[21] Teens may thus eschew familial world views (eg, religious beliefs, rituals, and values). After a death, grieving teens may find previously held religious beliefs challenged; similarly, those without prior faith may explore spirituality. Overall, grieving adolescents are greatly aided by finding other grieving teens, and family bereavement centers can be safe havens for peer support.

An informed child/adolescent psychiatrist or primary physician can normalize aspects of grief; anticipate symptoms of grief for clients/families; provide psychoeducation, support, and risk assessment throughout the tasks of grief across developmental stages; and remind families and clinicians not to over-pathologize grief in youth.

COMPLICATED GRIEF

Because many children and adolescents move toward integrated grief without professional intervention, it can be clinically challenging to know when to intervene or when to let grief travel its natural course. It becomes important, therefore, to resist the temptation to provide unnecessary therapy or medications and to develop skills to discern when grief warrants intervention.

Thoughts, emotions, and behaviors may arise during grief that (1) persist longer than expected by cultural norms and evidence-based expectations, (2) disrupt the natural progression from acute to integrated grief, and (3) become maladaptive. This extended and problematic process is called complicated grief (CG) or prolonged grief and requires intervention by the child/adolescent psychiatrist. CG is a term used by researchers for more than 20 years to describe grief that does not progress to integrated grief but becomes persistent and impairing instead. A similar entity is called prolonged grief disorder (PGD), a phrase that arose more recently in grief literature.[22] In the *Diagnostic and Statistical Manual of Mental Disorders* (Fifth Edition) (*DSM-5*), an entity called "Persistent Complex Bereavement Disorder" appeared in an effort to combine criteria and concepts from both CG and PGD. Although lack of consensus remains about precise terminology, there is recognition of an entity characterized by longer duration and severity than that found with acute grief and by impeded/delayed progression to integrated grief. The *DSM-5* definition and criteria include a shorter duration for extended grief symptoms in children than adults (6 months vs 12 months).

Complicated or prolonged grief is intense, turbulent, intrusive, prolonged, and maladaptive.[23] The term, *complicated*, is used in the medical sense—to indicate a process that impedes, slows, or complicates healing and integration. CG "is a distinct mental health disorder," and research indicates it affects 2% to 7% of the population.[15,16] Symptoms of CG or PGD include "intense yearning, longing, or emotional pain, frequent preoccupying thoughts and memories of the deceased person (or avoidance of such thoughts), a feeling of disbelief or an inability to accept the loss, and difficulty imagining a meaningful future without the deceased." It also includes deep sorrow, perseveration about details pertaining to the death, self-blame, feeling alone, feeling empty, or feeling that life has little purpose now.[15,16,22] Poor health outcomes are associated with CG in adults, including lower quality of life, cardiovascular disease and cancer, disrupted sleep, and suicidal ideation.[15,22] Research on CG has been conducted primarily with adults, but studies in children/adolescents show that young people also experience CG.[24] Familiarity with this entity is, therefore, paramount for clinicians.

Symptoms of complicated or prolonged grief must be distinguished from other comorbidities that impair functioning. Important distinctions exist among grief, major depressive disorder, and posttraumatic stress disorder (PTSD) (**Table 1**). If child and adolescent psychiatrists and pediatricians are aware of these differences, they will be better equipped to diagnose, guide, support, and recommend interventions for grieving patients. The adult literature reveals that a significant percentage of patients with bereavement-related depression also have CG. Likewise, among patients with CG, many experience depression.[15,16] It remains to be seen with further research if similar trends exist in children and adolescents.

ANTICIPATORY GRIEF/MOURNING

Anticipatory grief is a term coined in 1944 by Erich Lindemann,[17] a psychiatrist at Massachusetts General Hospital studying trauma-related grief after a historic fire in Boston, where many survivors with severe burns were treated at his hospital. Lindemann defined anticipatory grief as a response to the threat of death, rather than to death itself.

Table 1
Comparison of major depressive disorder, posttraumatic stress disorder, and complicated grief

Characteristic	Complicated Grief	Major Depression	Posttraumatic Stress Disorder
Affective symptoms			
Depressed mood (sadness)	Prominent, focused on the loss; core symptom	Prominent; diagnostic criterion	May be present
Anhedonia (loss of interest or pleasure)	Not usually present (and interest in thoughts of deceased is usually maintained)	Prominent and pervasive; diagnostic criterion	May be present
Anxiety	May be present, focused on loss and insecurity without the deceased	May be present	Prominent, focused on fear of recurrent danger; diagnostic criterion
Yearning or longing	Prominent, frequent, and intense; core symptom	Not usually present	Not usually present
Guilt	Common, focused on regrets related to the deceased	Usually present, related to feeling worthless and undeserving	May be present, focused on the traumatic event or its aftermath
Cognitive or behavioral symptoms			
Difficulty concentrating	May be present; not a core symptom	Common; diagnostic criterion	Common; diagnostic criterion
Preoccupying thoughts	Common, focused on thoughts and memories of the deceased; core symptom	May be present, focused on negative thoughts about self, others, or the world	Negative, exaggerated, distorted thoughts related to event; diagnostic criterion
Recurrent preoccupying images or thoughts	Common, focused on thoughts or memories of the deceased	May be present	Common, focused on event, usually associated with fear; diagnostic criterion

Avoidance of reminders of the loss	Common, focused on reminders of the finality of the loss and associated emotional distress	May be present, related to general social withdrawal	Common, focused on loss of sense of safety or reminders of event; diagnostic criterion
Seeking proximity to the deceased person	Common, focused on wanting to feel close to the deceased	Not usually present	Not usually present
Suicidal thinking and behaviors	Suicidal ideation often present; increased risk of suicidal behavior	Suicidal ideation present; diagnostic criterion; increased risk of suicidal behavior	Suicidal ideation present, increased risk of suicidal behavior
Abnormal eating behaviors	Avoiding certain foods or mealtimes to avoid reminders of the loss or eating favorite foods to feel close to the deceased	Change in eating due to change in appetite; diagnostic criterion	Not usually present
Sleep			
Disturbed sleep	Sleep disturbance related to avoiding bed or other reminders of the loss or rumination about troubling aspects of the death	Sleep disturbance common; diagnostic criterion	Sleep disturbance related to anxiety; diagnostic criterion
Nightmares	Not usually present	May be present	Related to the traumatic event; diagnostic criterion

From Shear MK. Complicated grief. N Engl J Med 2015;372(2):157; with permission.

Anticipatory grief is now understood to occur before an impending death.[18] It is experienced by loved ones and individuals facing their own impending death. It is distinct from grief that occurs after death, although there are shared features. Anticipatory grief not only focuses on future losses but also on past and present losses too. This combination differentiates it from post-loss grief: there is some rehearsal of death, attempts are made to accept death or adjust to its consequences before death occurs, and time remains to resolve issues and say goodbye. Grief scholar Therese Rando[25] advocates for the term, *anticipatory mourning*, versus anticipatory grief, arguing the former conveys a more complex experience that better represents the anticipatory process. In this article, the phrase "anticipatory grief" is used for simplicity's sake.

Relatives of a dying person can experience debilitating anticipatory grief, with resultant emotional confusion, hypervigilance, difficulty concentrating or making decisions, and sleep or appetite disruptions producing exhaustion. Anticipating the death of a child creates an unfathomable state for parents or siblings. During anticipatory grief, a person is in the present moment with an ill loved one, while simultaneously mourning both the person who existed in the past and the future the person will never enjoy. Anticipatory grief can engender similar emotional and physical symptoms as those from grief after death. Anticipatory grief cannot be stopped, fixed, or completely averted. A crucial role of the child/adolescent psychiatrist is to recognize, name, contain, and support the experience of anticipatory grief for those enduring it, which reassures them they are experiencing a known entity that others have endured before.

DISENFRANCHISED GRIEF

Kenneth J. Doka,[26] a scholar who has written extensively on disenfranchised grief for 30 years, defines this term as grief that "results when a person experiences a significant loss and the resultant grief is not openly acknowledged, socially validated, or publicly mourned. Disenfranchised grief is grief that is not culturally recognized. There is no social recognition that the person has a right to grieve, or "a claim for social sympathy or support."[26]

Examples of disenfranchised grief include grief after miscarriage or the death of a lover from an affair, the death of a partner from any culturally unsanctioned/unsupported relationship, or grief after the loss of physical integrity (eg, amputation or mastectomy). It may arise from multiple pregnancy losses or failure to conceive a child or for adolescent girls who have lost a pregnancy undisclosed to family members through miscarriage or elective termination. It may be grief over the death of an unknown biological parent. These and many other losses are sources of disenfranchised grief, and clinicians must consider this entity when younger patients present with emotional distress without verbalizing underlying etiology or appear to struggle with disclosure involving loss.

CHILDHOOD TRAUMATIC GRIEF

Bereaved children can develop a form of maladaptive grief associated with death-related trauma symptoms.[27] Judith Cohen, Anthony Mannarino, and Esther Deblinger[14] have researched extensively the treatment of children and trauma, and have written about the concept of childhood traumatic grief (CTG). They describe traumatic grief that develops after certain types of death/loss, including violent, accidental, sudden, and unexpected deaths (eg, from war, terrorism, suicide, homicide, and natural disasters). These can cause maladaptive patterns of grief and related cognitions and behaviors, wherein "both unresolved grief and PTSD symptoms are present, often accompanied by depressive symptoms as well."[14] These investigators caution that children and adolescents can also develop CTG after deaths/losses that may not be violent, sudden, or deemed "traumatic" by adults around them. One study of children and teenagers revealed that those who endured a parent's death after a lengthy illness "were more likely to develop PTSD and maladaptive grief symptoms than those who experienced the death of a parent due to sudden natural causes (eg, heart attacks)."[27] When treating youth with any history of grief or trauma, it is vital to remember these 2 entities may be linked, and trauma and grief may require separate treatment approaches to help the youth with CTG.

Cohen and colleagues[14] have developed a validated therapeutic intervention for CTG, called trauma-focused cognitive behavioral therapy (TF-CBT). Their research and that of others have demonstrated that TF-CBT interventions focused on trauma and CTG produce improvement in maladaptive and trauma-related symptoms. They recommend, however, that as a general rule, trauma issues should be addressed before grief issues can be appropriately navigated. They further note that CTG comprises a broader range of experiences and symptoms than the *DSM-5* entity Persistent Complex Bereavement Disorder. Children may develop CTG if they see or hear vivid images of a dying loved one's suffering or death if they also did not comprehend that person would die from his/her illness, of if they blame themselves for the death. Some children also develop somatic symptoms from the inability to process these experiences and negotiate the traditional tasks of mourning or grief.

GRIEF IN SOMATIC SYMPTOM AND CONVERSION DISORDERS

While assessing or treating children or teens with any of the types of grief described previously, psychiatrists may encounter significantly impairing physical symptomatology. Likewise, when observing somatic symptom or conversion disorder symptoms, psychiatrists may be sitting with a grieving youth. Somatic symptom and conversion disorders have been described for centuries, including in ancient Egyptian and Greek writings, and are increasingly common reasons for children and adolescents to see psychiatrists. Research from the 1980s and 1990s supports the concept that unresolved grief can cause conversion disorder in children and adolescents. In 1980, Michael Maloney[28] published a study exploring conversion reactions in 105 children and teens in which 54% had "unresolved grief reactions." Wolfelt[29] also noted that converted grief results in somatization and conversion reactions and called this a "grief avoidance response style," whereby the person unconsciously protects him/herself from the pain of loss and the psychological pain converts into physical symptoms. Lewis and Shonfeld[30], wrote that surviving children of deceased parents or siblings may develop conversion symptoms from identification with the dead loved one. Although this topic has not been extensively explored in recent literature and current research is required, it reminds clinicians to consider the possibility that grief may underlie a majority of somatic symptoms and conversion disorder presentations in youth. Addressing the grief may yield swifter resolution of impairing somatic symptoms in these conditions that historically have been difficult to treat.

TREATMENT INTERVENTIONS FOR GRIEF IN CHILDREN AND ADOLESCENTS

Death and its attendant losses are permanent. The death of a loved one cannot be reversed in the life of the child or adolescent who endures it. Because losses last a lifetime, grief can too. Grief does not disappear; rather, it ebbs, flows, lessens, and evolves over time but is not something young people necessarily get over or complete. As previously described, however, many children and adolescents traverse the tasks of mourning and find their way to integrated grief without professional assistance.[31]

The same is true of adults, and there is a body of literature on resilience that indicates it can be unproductive to introduce what Freud called "grief work" to a person when it is not needed.[32] For the smaller percentage of those who experience grief that significantly disrupts functioning in the months or years after a death, therapeutic interventions can facilitate more constructive coping and the road back toward integrated grief.

Bereavement counselors and family bereavement centers offering peer-support groups are excellent resources for families and youth experiencing the death of loved ones. These centers provide stabilizing support, education, processing space, and healing activities, and they provide a community of youth and families who understand, which mitigates the isolation so common in grieving youth. These centers often hold special events during holidays—Mother's Day, Father's Day, and so forth—which can help families navigate such moments in a supportive and safe environment. Agencies dedicated to specific diseases such as cancer and Alzheimer's disease, often provide support groups for bereaved families or for current caretakers enduring anticipatory grief. Child and adolescent psychiatrists may be called on to assess children/adolescents referred from these centers, from bereavement counselors, or from schools and pediatricians when grief appears complicated/prolonged or when it fails to respond to initial interventions. It is therefore important to maintain a list of local grief counselors, family bereavement centers or agencies, and related resources in one's region (eg, Compassionate Friends, community support groups, religious organizations, local bereavement counselors, and online resources). Child psychiatrists are further aided by knowing what interventions are empirically validated and what other therapeutic options might be clinically valuable.

Research has demonstrated that different psychotherapeutic interventions can be helpful in supporting a young person's grief. Among these, CG therapy (CGT) has been rigorously evaluated and found more effective than interpersonal therapy for CG/PG.[14] It is a structured course of weekly therapy focusing on resolving complications related to grief and supporting adaptation to the loss, with 2 main components: (1) restoration of function by finding enthusiasm and future planning and (2) integration of thoughts about the death that evoke less intense emotions, with incorporation of the loss and resumption of a meaningful life without the deceased person. Evidence supports allowing the bereaved person to tell and retell the story of the death, until it has been better incorporated and processed.[18] As previously discussed for CTG, TF-CBT is an evidence-based structured approach offered through training workshops and literature to guide the clinician in therapy, with 10 trauma-focused components and 4 grief-focused components.[14] Family-focused grief therapy (FFGT) is a form of family therapy specific to bereaved families in the palliative care setting and has shown modest positive outcomes in functioning for specific types of families.[33] For psychiatrists unable to obtain training in CGT, TF-CBT, or FFGT, or in whose region family bereavement centers are not available, other more generalized psychotherapeutic strategies will still prove valuable.

First and foremost, it is important for child psychiatrists and other clinicians to use active listening with grieving children and teens, and grant safe space in which they can tell and retell their stories of grief, until they feel the narrative is more integrated. Provide psychoeducation about grief, its symptomatology, and its unpredictability, duration, and uniqueness for each person. An important component of therapeutic interaction is to normalize grief experiences and provide reassurance youth are not going crazy (if they describe preoccupation with the deceased, talking to the deceased, distractibility, and so forth). Other strategies include: reassuring youth that the death was not their fault–this can be stabilizing and anxiety-reducing; encouraging parents to be transparent about the death circumstances and to let children attend funerals, with adequate support; helping youth identify their personal supports/circles so they know whom to call, text, and so forth when they need to talk or emote or want reassurance or guidance; reinforcing young patients' resilience and ability to tolerate their grief. Reinforce young patients' resilience and ability to tolerate their grief. Finally, helping youth identify which of Worden's tasks of mourning is most troublesome and providing support through the tasks of mourning can be useful.

Explore defenses mechanisms and positive and negative coping styles.[34] Differentiate depression from grief and provide anticipatory guidance about the potential for CG. Identify avoidance behaviors and teach youth to avoid avoidance (ie, there is no way through it but through it). Cognitive behavioral strategies to help grieving youth reframe negative cognitions (filtering, personalizing, catastrophizing, and so forth) can be extremely helpful, and reality testing or generating evidence for/against can assist with prevalent guilt. Work with children/teens to create coping skills toolboxes, including strategies for use when they feel overwhelmed (coping cards, emotion-regulation strategies or options, and so forth). Help children memorialize and retain connection to their loved ones through memory boxes, artwork, writing letters, keepsakes, or what Volkan[35] and others call "linking objects."[36] Recognize that death anniversaries, birthdays, holidays, special days such as Mother's Day, Father's Day, and graduations, may be triggering events for grief, and encourage youth or families to plan ahead as to whether/how they might observe these events, which will afford control and predictability. Connect youth to local or online family bereavement groups or community grief networks.

Clinicians can further participate in additional grief training online or through workshops/conferences; they can help develop grief curricula for professional students they supervise and can advocate at regional, state, and provincial levels for greater grief awareness for children, youth and families in schools, hospitals, health centers, and so forth

Psychiatric medications, such as selective serotonin reuptake inhibitors (SSRIs) and mirtazapine, may be beneficial primarily if there is comorbid depression, anxiety, insomnia, or poor appetite, or if a clinician is concerned about suicidal ideation from clinical depression. Research on psychopharmacology in grief is limited, and to date has largely involved adult subjects. Some evidence suggests that SSRIs can be helpful in both symptom relief and treatment adherence.[14,18] Benzodiazepines have not been found helpful, similar to findings in PTSD, where benzodiazepines are ineffective in improving outcomes. Given a lack of definitive data, the general approach in child and adolescent psychiatry—that of trialing therapy/counseling for a period of months prior to initiating medications—may prove the most prudent course. If evidence of significant suicidality, major depressive disorder, or impairing anxiety or panic symptoms exists, an SSRI trial should be more swiftly considered, based on clinical judgment and in accordance with standard best practices.

SUMMARY

As she was dying, Elizabeth Kübler-Ross reflected on her 5 stages of death and dying and recognized that the particular stages themselves and the order therein were not absolute. She wrote, "I now know that the purpose of my life is more than these stages...I have loved and lost, and I am so much more than five stages. And so are you."[1]

The work of child and adolescent psychiatrists, among other clinicians, in supporting youth who are grieving, extends beyond an earlier, 5-stage model of grief. Different professionals will have different training or skill levels in supporting grieving children and adolescents, and different community bereavement resources exist depending on practice location. In the context of this variability, child psychiatrists at minimum must seek education that allows them to differentiate the various forms of grief experienced by young patients and to offer useful interventions. The provision of active listening; psycho-education about grief—its physical, psychological, and spiritual effects; and the primary tasks of mourning, performance of risk assessment, and teaching of coping strategies are all important components of effective work with grieving children and families.

Because so little about grief is taught in medical school and residency, child and adolescent psychiatrists must attend to this knowledge gap in their own continuing medical education and in their teaching of trainees. Although education on death and dying and end-of-life communication is growing in the profession, it is not the same as education about grief, especially with youth. Advocacy and curricular devel-opment can ensure the next generation of medical professionals is adequately equip-ped to support grieving young patients and families. The Dougy Center (The National Center for Grieving Children & Families) in Oregon suggests to families that if a child needs help with grief due to impaired functioning after a death, the family should feel free to seek the advice of a qualified mental health professional and not be afraid "to ask about their experience and training in grief and loss, and their treatment phi-losophy and methods."[37] Child and adolescent psychiatrists, among other mental health clinicians, want to be prepared to respond to such queries with compassion, knowledge, and skill.

Grief may indeed be everywhere for children who have physical and/or psycholog-ical illness, yet medical providers do not always recognize or describe it as grief. Cli-nicians, educators and other providers who focus on whole-person and family-centered care will want to attend to childhood, adolescent and family grief by increasing the space and time within clinics, schools, and communities for children and teens to give voice to grief—both the nonpathologic and complicated/prolonged forms alike. They, and we, can serve as a powerful collective voice to increase grief literacy and resilience in patients, communities, schools, and society at large (**Box 1**).

Box 1
Selected resources for clinicians

Center for Complicated Grief at the Columbia University School of Social Work (www.complicatedgrief.org)

Compassionate Friends network (www.compassionatefriends.org)

The Dougy Center/The National Center for Grieving Children & Families (www.dougy.org)

National Alliance for Grieving Children (https://childrengrieve.org)

Olivia's House (www.Oliviashouse.org)

Winston's Wish (www.winstonswish.org.uk)—UK charity for bereaved children

www.Helpwithgrief.org

www.Griefspeaks.com

www.Griefnet.org

www.Centerforloss.com

Some clinical instruments used in adult grief assessments

Brief Grief Questionnaire

Inventory of Complicated Grief

Hogan Grief Inventory

Texas Revised Inventory of Grief

REFERENCES

1. Kübler-Ross E, Kessler D. On grief and grieving: finding the meaning of grief through the five stages of loss. New York: Scribner; 2005. p. xi–xii.
2. McCarthy JR. 'They all look as if they're coping, but I'm not': the relational power/lessness of 'youth' in responding to experiences of bereavement. J Youth Stud 2007;10(3):285–303.
3. Rosen R. Sheryl Sandberg's advice for grieving. The Atlantic.Com 2017. Available at: https://www.theatlantic.com/business/archive/2017/04/sandberg-optionb/524640/. Accessed October 20, 2017.
4. Kirwin K, Hamrin V. Decreasing the risk of complicated bereavement and future psychiatric disorders in children. J Child Adolesc Psychiatr Nurs 2005;18:62–78.
5. Harrison L, Harrington R. Adolescents' bereavement experiences. prevalence, association with depressive symptoms, and use of services. J Adolesc 2001; 24(2):159–69.
6. Torbic H. Children and grief: but what about the children? Home Healthc Nurse 2011;29(2):67–77.
7. Owens DA. Recognizing the needs of bereaved children in palliative care. J Hosp Palliat Nurs 2008;10(1):14–6.
8. Guldin M, Li J, Pedersen HS, et al. Incidence of suicide among persons who had a parent who died during their childhood. A population-based cohort study. JAMA Psychiatry 2015;72(12):1227–34.
9. Li J, Vestergaard M, Cnattingius S, et al. Mortality after parental death in childhood: a nationwide cohort study from three Nordic Countries. PLoS Med 2014; 11(7):1–13.
10. Grief in the Classroom: nationwide survey among school teachers on childhood bereavement. Conducted by the American Federation of Teachers and New York Life Foundation. 2012. Available at: https://www.aft.org/sites/default/files/release_bereavement121012.pdf. Accessed June 4, 2017.
11. Worden JW. Children and grief: when a parent dies. New York: Guilford Press; 2001. p. 11–6.
12. Wolfelt A. The journey through grief: the six needs of mourning. Fort Collins (CO): Center for Loss & Life Transition Publication; 2016. Available at: https://www.centerforloss.com/2016/12/journey-grief-six-needs-mourning/. Accessed June 4, 2017.
13. Rando TA. What therapists need to know about traumatic bereavement: what it is and how to approach it." Presented at: Lowcountry Mental Health Conference workshop. Charleston (SC). August 7, 2014. Available at: http://www.lowcountrymhconference.com/wp-content/uploads/2014/07/drrando_handout.pdf. Accessed May 29, 2017.
14. Cohen JA, Mannarino AP, Deblinger E. Treating trauma and traumatic grief in children and adolescents. New York: Guilford Publications; 2016. p. 16–20.
15. Shear KM. Complicated grief. N Engl J Med 2015;372(2):153–60.
16. Shear KM, Ghesquiere A, Glickman K. Bereavement and complicated grief. Curr Psychiatry Rep 2013;15(11):406.
17. Lindemann E. Symptomatology and management of acute grief. Am J Psychiatry 1944;101(2):141–8.
18. Simon NM. Treating complicated grief. JAMA 2013;310(4):416–23.
19. Bowlby J. Disruptions of affectional bonds and its effects on behavior. Contemp Psychother 1970;2:75.
20. Bowlby J. Attachment and loss: retrospect and prospect. American Journal of Orthopsychiatry 1982;52(4):664–78.

21. Piaget J, Inhelder B. The growth of logical thinking from childhood to adolescence: an essay on the construction of formal operational structures (Vol. 84). London: Routledge; 2013.
22. Prigerson HG, Horowitz MJ, Jacobs SC, et al. Prolonged grief disorder: psychometric validation of criteria proposed for DSM-V and ICD-11. PLoS Med 2009; 6(8):e1000121.
23. Horowitz MJ, Siegel B, Holen A, et al. Diagnostic criteria for complicated grief disorder. Focus 2003;1(3):290–8.
24. Melhem NM, Moritz G, Walker M, et al. Phenomenology and correlates of complicated grief in children and adolescents. J Am Acad Child Adolesc Psychiatry 2007;46(4):493–9.
25. Rando TA. Clinical dimensions of anticipatory mourning: theory and practice in working with the dying, their loved ones and their caregivers. Champaign (IL): Research Press; 2000. p. 1–98.
26. Doka KJ, editor. Disenfranchised grief: new directions, challenges, and strategies for practice. Research Press Pub; 2002. p. 7.
27. Kaplow JB, Howell KH, Layne CM. Do circumstances of the death matter? Identifying socioenvironmental risks for grief-related psychopathology in bereaved youth. J Trauma Stress 2014;27(1):42–9.
28. Maloney MJ. Diagnosing hysterical conversion reactions in children. J Pediatr 1980;97(6):1016–20.
29. Wolfelt AD. Toward an understanding of complicated grief: a comprehensive overview. Am J Hosp Palliat Care 1991;8(2):28–30.
30. Lewis M, Schonfeld DJ. Role of child and adolescent psychiatric consultation and liaison in assisting children and their families in dealing with death. Child Adolesc Psychiatr Clin North America 1994;3(3):613–27.
31. Silverman PR, Worden JW. Children's reactions in the early months after the death of a parent. Am J Orthopsychiatry 1992;62:93104.
32. Bonanno GA. The other side of sadness. What the new science of bereavement tells us about life after loss. New York: Basic Books; 2009.
33. Kissane DW, McKenzie M, Bloch S, et al. Family focused grief therapy: a randomized, controlled trial in palliative care and bereavement. Am J Psychiatry 2006; 163(7):1208–18.
34. Worden JW. Grief counseling and grief therapy: a handbook for the mental health practitioner. New York: Springer publishing Company; 2008.
35. Volkan VD. Linking objects and linking phenomena: a study of the forms, symptoms, metapsychology, and therapy of complicated mourning. New York: International Universities Press; 1981.
36. Wheeler I. The role of linking objects in parental bereavement. OMEGA-Journal of Death and Dying 1999;38(4):289–96.
37. "Tips for Supporting the Grieving Teen" The Dougy Center online resources. Available at: https://www.dougy.org/docs/TDC_Grieving_Teen_Tip_Sheet_2015. pdf. Accessed October 20, 2017.

The Medical Transition from Pediatric to Adult-Oriented Care
Considerations for Child and Adolescent Psychiatrists

Laura C. Hart, MD, MPH[a], Gary Maslow, MD, MPH[b],*

KEYWORDS

- Transition from pediatric to adult-oriented care • Transitional care
- Adolescent health • Continuity of care

KEY POINTS

- The transition from pediatric to adult-oriented care is a process, rather than simply the hand-off from a pediatric to an adult-oriented provider, and should take place in stages over the adolescent years.
- Guidelines and tools have been developed to assist providers in addressing the transitional care needs of adolescents and young adults.
- Child and adolescent psychiatrists play a particularly important role for those adolescents and young adults with primarily mental health needs, mental illness with onset in the adolescent and young adult period, and adolescents and young adults with intellectual and developmental disabilities.

BACKGROUND

The need for transitional care, care provided as teens and young adults move from the pediatric to adult-oriented health system, is in some ways among the success stories of medicine. In the last 50 years, improvements in pediatric care have turned previously fatal childhood illnesses into chronic and often manageable ones. Survival rates for cancer have improved dramatically.[1,2] Many complex congenital heart defects can be repaired or palliated.[3] Cystic fibrosis can be managed with appropriate treatment.[4]

Disclosure Statement: Nothing to disclose.
[a] Cecil G. Sheps Center for Health Services Research, University of North Carolina at Chapel Hill, 725 Martin Luther King Jr. Boulevard, Chapel Hill, NC, 27514, USA; [b] Psychiatry and Behavioral Sciences, Duke University School of Medicine, Durham, NC, USA
* Corresponding author. 2608 Erwin Road, Suite 300, Durham, NC 27705.
E-mail address: Gary.maslow@duke.edu

Child Adolesc Psychiatric Clin N Am 27 (2018) 125–132
http://dx.doi.org/10.1016/j.chc.2017.08.004
1056-4993/18/© 2017 Elsevier Inc. All rights reserved.

childpsych.theclinics.com

Adults with these diseases were rare even 20 or 30 years ago, and now there are 400,000 adult-aged survivors of pediatric cancers,[1] over 1 million adults with a congenital heart disease,[5] and as many adults who had cystic fibrosis as children.[6] Adolescents and young adults cared for primarily by a child and adolescent psychiatrist are particularly vulnerable during this time. Before considering the details of transitional care more fully, it is useful to remember that transition is a process to help a teen or young adult with chronic illness move into a future that their predecessors with similar issues never had the opportunity to experience.

It cannot be emphasized enough that transition is a process, and not simply the moment that care is handed off from the pediatric to the adult provider.[7] That handoff is more appropriately termed the transfer of care and should be a step in the larger transition process, which ideally also includes education for youth about their illness, the opportunity to practice and develop self-management and self-advocacy skills, and a move toward greater independence before transfer, as well as time to get settled with the appropriate adult-oriented provider after transfer.[8]

At present, many teens and young adults experience poor health outcomes around the time of transition and transfer, such as loss of control of diabetes[9] and problems with organ rejection in transplant recipients.[10] Teen and young adults with mental health conditions face similar challenges during transition. One study found that only 28% of young adults with a *Diagnostic and Statistical Manual of Mental Disorders*, fourth edition, diagnosis had received psychiatric care in the previous 3 months, whereas 50% of teens 12 to 17 years old had received care in the same timeframe.[11] In a prospective study in England, only 41 out of 154 young adults who were eligible for referral to adult mental health care were following long-term with adult-oriented mental health services.[12] In addition to less access to care, young adults also have higher rates of suicide than adolescents.[13]

BARRIERS

The barriers that are preventing more patients from getting effective transitional care have been well-documented. All of the parties involved in the transition process, including patients, parents, pediatric providers, and adult-oriented providers, have noted problems and concerns with the transition process. Patients find adult-oriented providers, clinics, and hospitals to be confusing to navigate and report feeling unsupported once they leave the pediatric setting.[14–16] Parents frequently report that providers address transition too late, leaving patients and families little time to consider all the needs of the transition process.[14,16–18] Pediatric providers cite a lack of time, training, and reimbursement for transition services as the major barriers of transitional care that they face.[19,20] Adult-oriented providers believe that they get little information from pediatric providers before seeing young adult patients and feel ill-equipped to provide care for young adults with pediatric-onset illnesses.[21,22] They also find that young adults lack the necessary knowledge and skills to manage their illness.[22]

The patient–doctor relationship presents another challenge in addressing transition effectively. Pediatric providers often become very close to the patients they care for and vice versa. Pediatric providers have often supported their patients and families through difficult medical and social problems. In some cases, a patient and her family may have been seeing the same doctor at regular intervals for the patient's entire life. When patients, parents, and pediatricians are faced with the difficult prospect of ending this years-long, strong, supportive relationship, all parties are understandably hesitant.[14,15,18] This hesitancy is probably part of the reason that only 40% of parents surveyed in the National Survey of Children with Special Health Care Needs reported addressing transition with a provider.[23,24] However, careful and thoughtful transition planning becomes all the more important in this situation. If pediatricians are hesitant to talk about transition in visits then, of course, parents will feel unprepared to leave pediatric care. If they do not clearly communicate to the next provider, then invariably that next provider will feel ill-equipped to care for that patient. If parents are not considering the steps a teenager must take to be more independent then, not surprisingly, the patient will be lacking in self-management skills. So, for teenagers and young adults with chronic illnesses, this understandable hesitancy to confront transition is not in the best interest of anyone, especially the patient. Pediatric providers seek to help patients become their best possible selves, and that must include addressing transition for adolescent and young adult patients.

GUIDELINES AND RESOURCES

Guidelines have been developed to help pediatric providers address transition in their practice. The most well-known guidelines regarding the transition from pediatric to adult-oriented care were jointly endorsed by the American Academy of Pediatrics (AAP), the American College of Physicians (ACP), and the American Academy of Family Physicians (AAFP), and published in *Pediatrics* in 2011.[8] Because there are no published guidelines specific to mental health transition, the AAP-ACP-AAFP guidelines serve as the best set of general guidelines from which to start considering the mental health transition process.

The AAP-ACP-AAFP guidelines recommend starting the transition process at the age of 12 years with an introduction to the transition process and the expected timeline over which transition and transfer are expected to happen. Starting transition in the early teen years lays the foundation on which future transition planning and education can build. As youth progress through the teenage years, the guidelines recommend evaluating a youth's transition readiness; that is, their ability to manage their illness, and developing a plan with patients and families to help patients build transition readiness skills, such as medication management. Providers can also facilitate transition readiness during visits by increasing youth engagement in visits, so that they can be more prepared for adult-oriented visits, in which they will be expected to take the lead in the encounter. Guidelines also emphasize the importance of a transfer letter to help adult-oriented providers obtain accurate easy-to-manage information about a new young adult patient. Existing providers are encouraged to ensure patients are established with new providers and to remain available to patients and new providers if questions arise after transfer.

Resources have been developed to assist patients, parents, and providers to address the needs of adolescent and young adults during the transition process. The most well-known of these is the Got Transition Web site (gottransition.org). For providers, Got Transition has taken the broad recommendations from the AAP-ACP-AAFP guidelines and converted them into processes and tools for practices to implement when they seek to improve their delivery of transitional care. The tools are centered on the Six Core Elements of Transition.[25,26] These are as follows:

1. Transition policy
2. Transition tracking and monitoring
3. Transition readiness
4. Transition planning
5. Transfer of care
6. Completion of transfer.

Each element includes specific steps for practices to implement as part of effective handling of the element. Within the transition policy element, for example, practices should develop a policy for transition, display that policy in public spaces in their offices, and ensure that all patients and families get a copy of the policy at age 12 to 13 years. Steps within the transition tracking element include establishing criteria the practice will use to identify the target population. The transition readiness element includes identifying a measure of transition readiness for use in practice and incorporating that measure into clinical practice. Steps within transition planning include establishing procedures to determine the need for decision-making support before the age of 18 years, as well as procedures to identify and communicate with the selected adult provider. The transfer of care element focuses on preparing and sending a transfer package with a brief but complete medical summary for accepting providers. The completion of transfer element includes following up with transferred patients and accepting providers after the first visit with the accepting provider to ensure that all questions have been addressed.

Previous studies have noted that providers believe they lack the time to have the previously described discussions with patients.[19,20] The developers of the tools from the Got Transition Web site have used a quality improvement approach to implement the Six Core Elements, and showed that using this approach did result in some improvements in the transition processes in the clinics involved.[27] It also provides a method for addressing some parts of transition, even if a clinician believes that he or she may not have the resources to address the entire process at a given time.

The guidelines and the Six Core Elements of transition were developed for primary care providers to use within patient-centered medical homes. Nonetheless, specialty societies have affirmed the importance of several of the principles and practices recommended here. For example, the consensus statement regarding the neurologist's role in transition reiterates the importance of early discussions, planning, and ensuring adult-oriented providers have been identified.[28] The guidelines for managing attention deficit hyperactivity disorder in the United Kingdom also emphasize the importance transition for that population, including youth and parent involvement in the transition process, and communication between pediatric and adult providers.[29]

SPECIAL CONSIDERATIONS FOR CHILD PSYCHIATRISTS

There are several specific transition scenarios that are particularly relevant to child and adolescent psychiatrists, including transitioning patients to college mental health services, treating youth with new onset psychosis during this vulnerable time period, and treating adolescent and young adults with intellectual or developmental disabilities (IDDs).

The full scope of college mental health is not discussed here; however, it is important to consider the transition to college as a period of vulnerability and to plan with patients and their families how to handle mental health care in a new setting. In particular, most colleges have robust mental health services and students can often access these without charge. It is important to have a plan for communicating with a patient as he or she transitions to college, and to make clear what care will be provided by the child and adolescent psychiatrist versus the college mental health service.[30] Having this discussion up front with patients is critical so that there is not confusion when they arrive at college.

Young adulthood is a period during which many major mental health disorders first present, including bipolar disorder and psychotic processes such as schizophrenia. Several studies have identified the unique vulnerability facing youth with new onset psychosis disorders and have highlighted the need for organized transition services to ensure that these youth stay in care.[31–33] It is important for them to stay in care to prevent noncompliance, which can result in worsening symptoms and potentially worse long-term outcomes. Following the Got Transition core elements approach to this special population could be an effective way for a child and adolescent psychiatry practice to keep track of their most vulnerable patients and ensure a smooth transition to adult care.

Many child and adolescent psychiatrists provide care for children, adolescents, and young adults with IDD, including individuals with autism. There are many unique considerations when planning the medical transition for such individuals. In particular, if there is significant intellectual disability, there is a need for establishing supportive decision-making, often including full guardianship at the time the youth turns 18 years old. For child and adolescent psychiatry practices, establishing clear guidelines for clarifying decision-making status and guardianship is critical in discussions with families as they help their child navigate complex health care and community services.[34] Johnson[34] wrote a review of the challenges facing young adults with intellectual disability and identified 3 processes that must occur simultaneously: "(1) from child- and family-centered pediatric care to adult-oriented health care, (2) from school environment to work place, and (3) from home to community."[34] Child and adolescent psychiatrists can play a key role in supporting young adults with IDD, and their parents, as they navigate these complex transitions.

Beyond the general recommendations previously described, the authors offer a couple of pro tips to child psychiatrists as they treat adolescents and young adults during their transition to adult-oriented care.

Pro Tip 1: Do Not Assume Patients Are Following Up with Other Providers

Studies have shown that teens may stop seeing their specialty providers well before they are ready to transfer. In a study of patients with congenital heart disease, approximately 47% of patients with congenital heart disease were no longer following with a cardiologist regularly by the age of 17 years.[35] In the authors' experience, almost 40% of youth with chronic illnesses ranging from type 1 diabetes to sickle cell disease to inflammatory bowel were lost to follow-up before transfer to an adult-oriented provider.[36] Given the high proportions of patients who stop following with their providers, a patient who is following with a provider cannot be assumed to be following with others. As such, a key component of the role of the child psychiatrist treating medically complex patients is to ensure that these patients continue to follow-up with the other pediatric providers involved in their care, which will help facilitate a more effective transition for the patient.

Pro Tip 2: Try to Coordinate Transition Efforts with Patients' Other Providers

Just as patients may not be seeing other providers, they may also be seeing several, particularly patients with concomitant complex medical and mental health concerns. Although all providers need to assist in their patients' transition process, coordination among providers can help to streamline the transition process for patients and families.

If a provider has identified the appropriate mental health providers for a patient, she or he should communicate the names and contact information for these new providers to a patient's other pediatric providers, especially the provider who is coordinating the transition, whether that is the patient's primary care provider or a particular specialist. Ideally, the provider who is coordinating the transition can then include the name of the accepting mental health providers for the accepting medical providers to ensure coordination within the new adult-oriented care team.

Pro Tip 3: Aim to Have Transfer Occur During a Time of Stability

This tip is not necessarily unique to child psychiatrists but does deserve special consideration in the context of transition for teenagers and young adults with mental health concerns. If a young person is transferred while in the middle of a recurrence of major depression, for example, that young person is being asked to arrange for care with new providers, to meet them, and to become comfortable with them while also facing significant symptoms. It is a lot to ask. By transferring during a time of stability, patients are given the necessary time to become comfortable with their new mental health providers before, rather than during, a crisis. Circumstances do not always allow for this smooth hand-off while things are going well but, when they do, capitalizing on this opportunity pays great dividends.

SUMMARY

The transition from pediatric to adult-oriented care continues to present challenges to patients, parents, and providers alike. Nonetheless, it is an important step in ensuring the success of teens and young adults as they move toward greater independence. Guidelines provide recommendations to providers, and resources are available for providers to use in implementing improved transition processes. Child psychiatrists play an important role in supporting teens and young adults with mental health concerns during transition. The authors encourage providers to proactively support their teenage and young adult patients as they leave the pediatric health system and enter adult-oriented care.

REFERENCES

1. Childhood cancer survivor study: an overview. Available at: www.cancer.gov/types/childhood-cancers/ccss. Accessed September 8, 2016.
2. Hunger SP, Lu X, Devidas M, et al. Improved survival for children and adolescents with acute lymphoblastic leukemia between 1990 and 2005: a report from the children's oncology group. J Clin Oncol 2012;30(14):1663–9.
3. Said SM, Driscoll DJ, Dearani JA. Transition of care in congenital heart disease from pediatrics to adulthood. Semin Pediatr Surg 2015;24(2):69–72.
4. Flume PA, O'sullivan BP, Robinson KA, et al. Cystic fibrosis pulmonary guidelines: chronic medications for maintenance of lung health. Am J Respir Crit Care Med 2007;176(10):957–69.
5. van der Bom T, Zomer AC, Zwinderman AH, et al. The changing epidemiology of congenital heart disease. Nat Rev Cardiol 2011;8(1):50–60.
6. About cystic fibrosis. Available at: www.cff.org/What-is-CF/About-Cystic-Fibrosis/. Accessed September 8, 2016.
7. Blum RW, Garell D, Hodgman CH, et al. Transition from child-centered to adult health-care systems for adolescents with chronic conditions. A position paper of the Society for Adolescent Medicine. J Adolesc Health 1993;14(7):570–6.
8. Cooley WC, Sagerman PJ. Supporting the health care transition from adolescence to adulthood in the medical home. Pediatrics 2011;128(1):182–200.
9. Nakhla M, Daneman D, To T, et al. Transition to adult care for youths with diabetes mellitus: findings from a Universal Health Care System. Pediatrics 2009;124(6): e1134–41.

10. Watson AR. Non-compliance and transfer from paediatric to adult transplant unit. Pediatr Nephrol 2000;14(6):469–72.

11. Copeland WE, Shanahan L, Davis M, et al. Untreated psychiatric cases increase during the transition to adulthood. Psychiatr Serv 2015;66(4):397.

12. Singh SP, Paul M, Ford T, et al. Transitions of care from child and adolescent mental health services to adult mental health services (TRACK study): a study of protocols in Greater London. BMC Health Serv Res 2008;8(1):135.

13. Park MJ, Scott JT, Adams SH, et al. Adolescent and young adult health in the United States in the past decade: little improvement and young adults remain worse off than adolescents. J Adolesc Health 2014;55(1):3–16.

14. Gray WN, Resmini AR, Baker KD, et al. Concerns, barriers, and recommendations to improve transition from pediatric to adult IBD care: perspectives of patients, parents, and health professionals. Inflamm Bowel Dis 2015;21(7):1641–51.

15. Cheak-Zamora NC, Teti M. "You think it's hard now... It gets much harder for our children": youth with autism and their caregiver's perspectives of health care transition services. Autism 2015;19(8):992–1001.

16. DiFazio RL, Harris M, Vessey JA, et al. Opportunities lost and found: experiences of patients with cerebral palsy and their parents transitioning from pediatric to adult healthcare. J Pediatr Rehabil Med 2014;7(1):17–31.

17. Doyle M, Werner-Lin A. That eagle covering me: transitioning and connected autonomy for emerging adults with cystinosis. Pediatr Nephrol 2015;30(2):281–91.

18. Lochridge J, Wolff J, Oliva M, et al. Perceptions of solid organ transplant recipients regarding self-care management and transitioning. Pediatr Nurs 2013;39(2): 81–9.

19. American Academy of Pediatrics. Department of Research. Survey: transition services lacking for teens with special needs. AAP News 2009;30(11):12.

20. Geenen SJ, Powers LE, Sells W. Understanding the role of health care providers during the transition of adolescents with disabilities and special health care needs. J Adolesc Health 2003;32(3):225–33.

21. Okumura MJ, Kerr EA, Cabana MD, et al. Physician views on barriers to primary care for young adults with childhood-onset chronic disease. Pediatrics 2010; 125(4):e748–54.

22. Wright EK, Williams J, Andrews JM, et al. Perspectives of paediatric and adult gastroenterologists on transfer and transition care of adolescents with inflammatory bowel disease. Intern Med J 2014;44(5):490–6.

23. Lotstein DS, McPherson M, Strickland B, et al. Transition planning for youth with special health care needs: results from the National Survey of Children with Special Health Care Needs. Pediatrics 2005;115(6):1562–8.

24. Lotstein DS, Ghandour R, Cash A, et al. Planning for health care transitions: results from the 2005–2006 National Survey of Children With Special Health Care Needs. Pediatrics 2009;123(1):e145–52.

25. GotTransition. Resources for providers. Available at: http://www.gottransition.org/providers/index.cfm. Accessed September 8, 2016.

26. GotTransition. Guide for transition youth to adult health care providers. Available at: http://www.gottransition.org/providers/leaving.cfm. Accessed September 8, 2016.

27. McManus M, White P, Barbour A, et al. Pediatric to adult transition: a quality improvement model for primary care. J Adolesc Health 2015;56(1):73–8.

28. Brown LW, Camfield P, Capers M, et al. The neurologist's role in supporting transition to adult health care: a consensus statement. Neurology 2016;87(8):835–40.

29. National Collaborating Centre for Mental Health. National Institute for Health and Clinical Excellence: Guidance. Attention deficit hyperactivity disorder: diagnosis and management of ADHD in children, young people and adults. Leicester (United Kingdom): British Psychological Society (UK) The British Psychological Society & The Royal College of Psychiatrists; 2009.
30. Pedrelli P, Nyer M, Yeung A, et al. College students: mental health problems and treatment considerations. Acad Psychiatry 2015;39(5):503–11.
31. Malla A, Iyer S, McGorry P, et al. From early intervention in psychosis to youth mental health reform: a review of the evolution and transformation of mental health services for young people. Soc Psychiatry Psychiatr Epidemiol 2016; 51(3):319–26.
32. Birchwood M, Connor C, Lester H, et al. Reducing duration of untreated psychosis: care pathways to early intervention in psychosis services. Br J Psychiatry 2013;203(1):58–64.
33. Birchwood M, Lester H, McCarthy L, et al. The UK national evaluation of the development and impact of Early Intervention Services (the National EDEN studies): study rationale, design and baseline characteristics. Early Interv Psychiatry 2014;8(1):59–67.
34. Johnson CP. Transition into adulthood. Pediatr Ann 1995;24(5):268–73.
35. Mackie AS, Ionescu-Ittu R, Therrien J, et al. Children and adults with congenital heart disease lost to follow-up. Circulation 2009;120(4):302–9.
36. Hart L, Chung R, Brown A, et al. Clinic utilization in youth and young adults with chronic illness around the time of expected transfer to adult-oriented care. Poster Presentation presented at Society of General Internal Medicine. Hollywood, FL, May 13, 2016.

Printed and bound by CPI Group (UK) Ltd, Croydon, CR0 4YY

03/10/2024

01040395-0014